# Substance Use
# DISORDER

## The Nightmare Brain Disease
## Killing Our Kids and Destroying Families

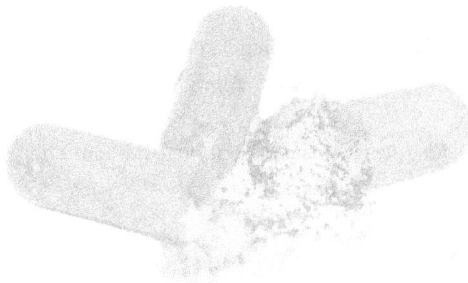

# Veronica Lazarus, MD, MS, MA

For information regarding special discounts for bulk purchases, please contact the publisher:

LaBoo Publishing Enterprise, LLC
staff@laboopublishing.com

# Contents

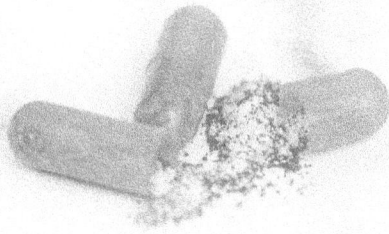

# Introduction

One week before I embarked on this writing project, I heard a story on the news about a young, distraught mother who was explaining with great pain how her fourteen-year-old son went to bed in his room and never woke up. She ended her painful interview asking a critical question: Why didn't anyone tell the parents about the dangers of drug death that could suddenly take her beautiful, curious son away? On hearing this painful story for the third time, I realized that I, as a physician, could no longer stay silent. I needed to share my own story about my son who has substance use disorder and the struggle it is to keep him alive. I wanted to help parents like myself, and I needed to do it now.

This book is written to tell the story about what I've learned from my son's suffering, and his family's suffering and to help the parents and families of America to better understand the dynamics of Substance Use Disorder and the damage being done to families and the American workforce.

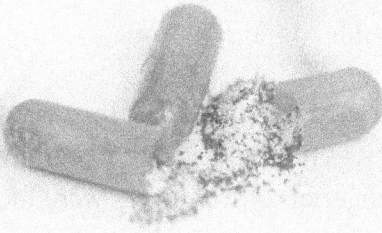

# Chapter 1

I was born the first of nine children in Lagos, West Africa. My parents were very grounded and hardworking. My father, a civil engineer, and my mother ran a small business together that grew to become a larger business, and it provided the ability for my parents to build their own homes from the ground up. At that time, nobody gave anyone a loan from the bank. My father was from the Igbo tribe, and my mother was a combination of the Yoruba tribe and the Igbo tribe. My mother's family were society people and had a name that was recognized everywhere. Parents sent their girls to my grandmother's finishing school to learn etiquette, how to be young women, and how to talk properly, how to live, how to posture themselves, and how to make their own clothes as well as start a business as a seamstress. In those days, it was called home economics. The students were learning how to live better and carry themselves with dignity and to have elevated standards. I grew up learning to make dresses for my siblings with my mother and grandmother. My childhood was happy and responsible. I was raised to see life with great respect for God and people, especially people who were older than myself.

In 1967, the Biafran War started. The Ibos wanted to create their own country, as they believed that their lives would be better. Most of Nigerian oil resources were located in that part of the country. Because of the war, we moved from Lagos to Ibadan and then to Enugu, the capital of Enugu State in the eastern part of Nigeria, where my father's village was located. As soon as we arrived in the village, I was sent to grade school in Onitsha. This was during the early phase of the Biafran War.

At the Onitsha grade school, I quickly became friends with the younger sister of the wife of the then president and head of state of Biafra. The president's wife told me I didn't have to travel back and forth to my parents in the village because I could live with them during the school year. The president's wife was from my village as well.

I was in my early teens at the time. My friend and I were carefree and would do everything together. We moved to one of the state houses where the president's wife lived with his kids. In those days, we were ferried around in luxury. She had an American Chevy Impala with the license plate that said, "Impala 1." My teenage years in Onitsha were brief but interesting.

As time went on, the war got fiercer. There were bombings, and all the children at the school had to go back to the village to hide in the underground bunkers. I remember one morning when the bombing was so fierce and me and my siblings went down into the bunker to hide. We quickly discovered there were two snakes in the bunker. I was the first one who went down into the bunker, but when I saw the snakes, I ran like I'd never ran before. From that day forward, I refused to get back into the bunker. Like many people, I was afraid of snakes, and these were fairly large black snakes. I could not say what type of snakes they were. For all I knew, they could have been black mambas. I just wanted to get as far away as possible. The snake did not follow us or anything like that, and no one was bitten. Despite the bombing, I was willing to stay out of the bunker rather than go back and meet the snakes again.

I was the firstborn, so I was taught early that my responsibilities were in the care of my family and helping my parents with my siblings. I would ride my bike about fifteen miles to the market to get food for my family. Life during the war in Okporo was without basic need. You had to walk about two miles to the stream to get water. There was no electricity, so you had to fetch firewood, and everyone cooked outside. I occupied myself with reading. I read all of the plays of Shakespeare. I read whatever book I could lay my hands on. I knew I wanted to be somebody and to service people who were in need. I knew I wanted to be a medical doctor. Nothing was going to stop me, not even the war or poverty.

As the war raged, my father became involved in the war efforts of Biafra. As an engineer, he helped build the weapons needed in the war response. The opposition, the rest of Nigeria, was well funded, and the British did not agree that Nigeria should be split up. So they helped the opposition with whatever they needed to win the war and keep

Nigeria together as one country. It was in their best interest. By the grace of God, we all survived the war.

When the war was over in 1970, and Nigeria won, we returned to the western part of Nigeria to Lagos briefly then to Ibadan, where my parents were still building their home. I went back to finish grade school and went on to boarding school.

I got accepted to attend St. Anne's School in Ibadan, which was regarded as one of the best girls' schools in Nigeria and I believe in Africa in those days. I quickly excelled, and I became the head girl at the elite boarding school. Unlike the other girls' school, it was a private church school, and the standards were high. It was modeled around the English Church boarding school. The teachers would come from the United Kingdom. The principal was an English woman who loved Africa. A lot of the premier women of my age went to St. Anne's, and most of them had done well. I was shuttled between Ibadan and Lagos to spend holidays with my uncle, who was then the permanent secretary of economics for Nigeria and lived in a large lake-front house in Ikoyi, Lagos. Ms. Groves, the principal at St. Anne's, was very vested in girls' education. We had to learn languages, like French, and participated in sports, mostly track. She was portly built herself but followed a very rigid curriculum. It was a good time in my life, and all the girls I went to school with excelled and continued into higher education.

The school life at St. Anne's was particularly good. Ms. Groves was very English in her ways. She enjoyed living in Africa, and she would teach the girls proper English manners, the proper English way of handling difficulties, and everybody did well. She made sure we had books sent to us from the UK, and we lacked nothing for academics. So when I was appointed to become the head girl, I was very honored, and I took my job as a head girl at boarding school very seriously. It was during this time when I realized that I wanted to continue my education in America, not Britain. So I applied to different colleges and universities in America.

My aunt lived in the UK and was studying to be a nurse. I had read about everything American I could lay my hands on, and I had some idea that I could be a doctor if I went to America. To my knowledge, there were more challenges in the UK to become a doctor, as you had to study for a long time and the grammar school exam was really a tall order. At the time, America had been marketed as a great place to go to school. It had colleges in every state. I went to the market to find places I could use typewriters to complete my applications for the colleges. I applied and took my exam for English as a Foreign Language and the required exams to get into college. I did well enough and started receiving all types of letters from many schools that wanted me to come to their school. Then the package from University at Buffalo came and with it a host family that would help me adjust to life in America. I decided to accept the offer to go to the school in Buffalo, New York.

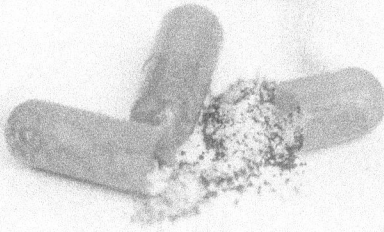

# Chapter 2

I was about 20 years old when I arrived in New York City with one suitcase in my hand. The taxi took me from the JFK Airport to where I would be staying at the Hotel Tudor near Grand Central Station. The Hotel Tudor was built in 1930 and had gone through many changes over the years, but when I was there, it was still mid luxury and modest.

New York City at the time was everything I had read about. With long, tall buildings and many cars. This was Manhattan, there was a lot of bustling activities, and it was not like any place I had seen before, except in pictures. I arrived in the city in the late afternoon and soon the lights were on everywhere. I had no idea where I was. My plan was to stay the night and then take a bus to Buffalo where I would meet the host family. The Hotel Tudor was in the Tudor City neighborhood of Manhattan, a historic district that boasted with Tudor-style architecture. The hotel itself was a higher-grade hotel, and at the time of this writing is known as the Westgate New York Grand Central. I was given a room with one bed, and I remember the lighting was low, but I could still see my way in the room. I did not leave the room until it was time for me to go catch my bus to Buffalo.

The next morning, after a 10-hour bus ride, I was met at the bus station by Mrs. Bozer, who with her husband and family became my host family. They had four kids of their own. They were some of the greatest human beings I have ever met. A great conservative Republican family. Dr. Bozer was a cardiologist, and his wife was an activist and a political director on women's voting rights.

When the oldest of the Bozer boys finished school at Harvard University in Cambridge, Massachusetts, he headed off to Africa and Nigeria was where he decided to explore. He spent time with my parents for a few months and got to know them. So it became a really solid relationship with the Bozer family and my family in Nigeria. How we long for those good, old days in America again, when people respected each other and trusted each other and there wasn't as much political divide and mistrust.

I finished my undergraduate education at SUNY Buffalo in four years with a bachelor arts/science in Biochemistry. Then I went to Boston and attended Northeastern for graduate school where I was studying pathology. I roomed with my schoolmate from grade school at St. Anne's, Ibadan, while she was studying at MIT. Ngozi Okonjo-Iweala has gone on to do great things, just like all the students who went to St. Anne's school—they were all very accomplished. She became the two-time Finance Minister of Nigeria and went on to the Brooklyn Institute in Washington, DC.

Before she finished in Nigeria, she helped Nigeria nego-
tiate its debt with the Paris Club and refinance the big
loans with interest that were weighing the country down.
So, when she finished, she went back to Brooklyn Institute
from where she was appointed in 2021 by the Biden administration to become Director-General of the World
Trade Organization.

I spent three years in Boston 1977-1980 and did graduate work at Northeastern and transferred back to the
University at Buffalo to complete my master's degree in pathology at SUNY Roswell Park. Still pursuing medicine, I
embarked in further graduate work at the medical school
in the hopes of getting a PhD in anatomy. In the Anatomy
department, I was privileged to work with Dr. Frances
Sansone and Dr. Harold Brody. I went back to Buffalo to
continue graduate school. I had to because my interest was
ultimately to study medicine. When I got back to Buffalo,
I enrolled with the anatomy department and became a
teaching assistant for anatomy and histology as a graduate
student. I loved anatomy and did so well that Dr. Harold
Brody, then the Chairman of Anatomy, recommended that
I study medicine and recommended me to the admission
board, and I went on to complete medical school in record
time. When I finished, I went on to do an internship for
internal medicine at the Buffalo General Hospital.

When the UCLA School of Medicine invited me to interview for a dermatology residency, I saw it as an opportunity
to move west and leave the Buffalo weather behind me. My
internship at Buffalo General Hospital was really hard. As

soon as I received that invitation, I went down to the Jeep dealership and picked up a brand-new Jeep Cherokee to drive across the country. I wanted to feel that air in my hair. I was alone and was not afraid. Sometimes I encountered strange truck drivers who would try to run me off the road as they saw I was alone in the vehicle. I would pull off the road at night, as I did not want to take any chances. I left my lovely Victorian home for my sister and her husband, who is also a doctor from the medical program in Buffalo. He did his undergraduate at Columbia in New York and enrolled in medical school in Buffalo where he met and married my sister. A very brilliant man. I was glad at that time to leave Buffalo for new experiences in academics in the west. I was not prepared for the politics and educational inequity in the West. I always thought the West would be more progressive, but the high institutions were the very bed of racial educational and health inequity in America.

In the fall of 1985, on arrival at UCLA, the British Dermatologist and Associate Professor of Dermatology, Dr. Lowe, who had never seen any person of color at the UCLA was determined to try to give me a spot in dermatology. He thought that if I were in everyone's face, I would get in because I was already there and had met all the qualifications and would also have published with him. When I got to UCLA, Dr. Nicholas Lowe pushed me into doing some clinical research with him. After two years of working in clinical research, I got a position that was nonpaid that he'd designed for me. I published some papers with him and presented my work at the annual American Academy of Dermatology Meeting and at the Annual meeting of the

Society of Investigative Dermatology. I received an award from the Society for my work. I was very thankful that somebody acknowledged my hard work, and my time and effort would not just be swept under the rug by people who had political agendas and racial, evil minds.

Shortly after this award, I decided to complete my residency in internal medicine, so I enrolled at UCLA Wadsworth, VA. After a year, a spot opened up at the UCI Long Beach, VA program. So I went from the UCLA program at Wadsworth to the UCI program at Long Beach. There I completed the residency in internal medicine.

In the two years at UCLA Dermatology, I focused and learned everything I needed to learn in clinical dermatology. Every day, I would travel from where I lived in the valley to UCLA and study with the dermatopathologist. He was a great guy, and he taught me as much as I wanted to learn. I would shadow Dr. Lowe to see the patients with clinical dermatology problems. I would shadow all the other dermatology attendings, and I learned so much, even surgical dermatology and flap repairs.

These surgical skills came in handy on one medical missionary trip to Sierra Leone. There was a middle-aged woman with fungating carcinoma of the left breast that was oozing and smelling. This woman's suffering was brought to our attention during the medical mission. There were two other medical doctors, a pediatrician, Dr. Robert Hamilton, and a cardiologist, Dr. Lawrence Czar. We also had a highly trained university nurse. We had no choice but to try to help the woman, by the grace of God. We had not planned to see any surgical problems. Usually on these medical missions, we encountered the garden routine variety problems. But this woman needed help, and we needed to do what we could do to help her feel better. After talking with the other doctors, it was clear they were not able to take on surgical intervention. There was no surgical suit or electricity, and there was no real anesthetic. We had a sterile set up; many bottles of lidocaine with epinephrine and ones without epinephrine. The nurse said she would help me, and we set up as best as we could. We prayed as we never prayed, and we went to work.

We cleaned the patient up and injected the lidocaine. I began to surgically excise the tumor that was open and draining around her left breast nipple. Some of the lesions were fixed to her chest wall. For hours we worked. On exam we noted that she also had large axillary lymph nodes that were hard and evidence of axillary node metastasis. When I was done removing and cleaning out the cancerous tumor, I noticed a defect and open chest wall lesion of four centimeters by six centimeters. To help you understand, a breast surgeon would normally require a full operating room staff to even attempt a surgery like this. This was a radical mastectomy with axillary nodes dissection under local anesthesia with a flashlight, in the dark on a church school table. I did not know if she would survive the procedure.

After that experience, I knew that we served a God that is very alive and very present in the daily affairs of human beings. The Lord can use anyone. How did I close a big opening left by this surgery? What I learned from my training at UCLA was what enabled me to help this woman. I borrowed skin from her abdomen, keeping the blood supply to the skin, and flipped it into the defect to close the wound. I thought she would not be able to get up from the surgery. I was exhausted, the nurse was exhausted, and I believe the other doctors were just praying for us. We closed her up and applied some drains and pressure, and she survived only by the grace of Jesus Christ. I serve a God who in darkness reveals His light.

The woman sat up and was thanking us for the surgery. She was in no pain, an even greater miracle. The double miracle was that everyone in her village who knew of her suffering and heard about the surgery came to accept Jesus Christ. I was most humbled that the Lord is always using the stones that the builders reject. We continued to monitor her until we left the country. When we returned to Los Angeles, St. John's Hospital in Santa Monica, who had been most amazingly helpful, gave us anti-cancer drugs to send back to Sierra Leone to be given to the woman by the local doctors we met there. Sometimes the Lord will use feeble hands to accomplish His greater purpose. It was the eternal soul of those people that the Lord was about, not our skill or great ability. We were tools in the hand of a Mighty God. We were also able to continue sending supplies to the local hospital to try to get it working again as there was no supply in the hospitals in 1993 in Junction Town, Freetown.

In 1990, I purchased a private practice in Santa Monica in the notable 2001 Building by St, John's Hospital. The practice used to have two physicians who had big celebrity clients. One was Elizabeth Taylor, though I never saw her myself, but there were many big-name celebrities in the practice I saw as a solo practitioner.

I went into product development to help booster my practice because my practice was a combination of internal medicine and dermatology. The product division had created over three hundred different products and sold them to other dermatologists and plastic surgeons across the nation. Most of the products that I developed were over-the-counter skin products.

In 1994, the Rwanda crisis was headline news and was hard to watch. There was so much suffering of the innocent children with cholera and malnutrition. So my office began to call emergency room doctors across the city. Everyone wanted to help. The ones who could not go donated money to help. Within one week, we had over thirty medical personnel ready and willing to go to Rwanda. By the following week, there were over thirty-seven medical personnel. We were now a group of our own.

When Doctors Without Borders would not take us, we called the United Nations. The United Nations High Commission on Refugees (UNHCR) took us in and provided the umbrella and cover we needed to proceed to the front line. Once we had that, it was like the flood gates opened for resources for our relief work. The Continental Airline provided us with seats on their flight to Germany. The US government chipped in and gave us a C17 with pallets of water and Meals Ready to Eat (MRE) to carry us to Goma Airport. I take this opportunity to thank them again because they were great men and women with compassion for their fellow human being. Their role was critical to that relief effort and established us as a foundation with 501c status at the time.

My practice was at the very forefront of global relief work with the likes of World Vision, Samaritan Purse, CARE, International Medical Corp, and many more. We were the new kids on the block at the time, but now we are twenty-seven years old in global relief work. We have never asked for any grant, yet we know that our work is greatly needed, especially now in the area of substance use disorder. Doctors and Nurses to the World Foundation could be that missing link for many new organizations that want to help in this crisis. We have global experience and global knowledge, as well as a globally recognized name.

When the US military took us to Goma Air Base, they could go no further, as the aircraft was really large and the only airbase in Zaire capable of landing it. Again, the United Nations gave us two smaller aircrafts to take us into Bukavu in Zaire under the umbrella of the United Nation High Commissioner Refugees where we had been assigned to work.

We thought we were going to be there for two weeks, but I ended up staying there for five and a half months. My two sons were too young to go with me, so they stayed at our home in Pacific Palisades with my husband, and my mother moved in to help take care of them while I was working in the bush in Bukavu. The tragedy and the smell of death was everywhere. Many kids died on the road from Rwanda to Zaire and Burundi. We quickly had to set up a tent hospital. The experience of being part of this global crisis in Rwanda was very life defining for me, and I'm sure for all the people who went with us.

From that experience, I was committed and made up my mind that I would continue to do medical relief, to help continue to serve people as a physician, while I tried to also provide for my family. When I was nine years old, I told my parents that I would study medicine and I would take care of the poor. The time I spent in Rwanda was an activation of that vision, and my life had purpose greater than myself and was in the service of God and helping my fellow human being. I am fulfilled. I never thought the road would be easy. However, there was never any self-focused intent in anything I did, ever since I could remember my life way back.

I had two sons, Jacques and Matthew, who were six years apart. When Jacques was old enough, he went on all the trips for medical missions with me, and he was very good at it. He enjoyed helping people. He would be the one running the pharmacy. We went to South America, in Guatemala and in Nicaragua. We were in West Africa, Gambia, Sierra Leone, Nigeria, and in the United States we were in Louisiana after Hurricane Katrina with medical personnel to help out.

One summer before going off to high school, my son kept talking about football. He was really good at it; from the time he was eight years old, he loved football. So when we sent him off to the famous Harrow School, which was a very elite grammar school in England that was founded in 1572, he was not happy to spend the summer there. He did not want to continue his education in the UK. He wanted to come back to United States and play American football.

That summer at Harrow was my son's first time at being on his own and meeting people from every culture. He was 14 years old. He liked a girl from Korea, and they hit it off really well. She was fourteen years old. I called the girl's family, as I could not understand them being so involved at such a young age with parents so far away. I was concerned for the girl. When the summer was over, my son just wanted to come back and play football. Nothing was more important to him.

My son had started his academics at the Lighthouse Academy. He was playing football there, but he felt that he had more talent and he wanted to go to a public school and on to a bigger college with a bigger football program. He also felt that he wasn't getting any playing time at the Church Academy football. Nobody said he couldn't go, so he started at Malibu High School and then he subsequently transferred to Pacific Palisades High.

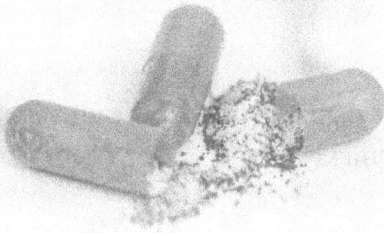

# Chapter 3

J acques had a lot of success when he was at Pacific Palisades High School on the football team. He was the top running back with his friend as quarterback and another of their friends as the receiver. They did very well. They were written up in the paper, and they were highly recruited by the colleges and universities. When UCLA came to recruit my son, they didn't want him to continue playing as the running back. He had many sport injuries because he had a tall, thin frame. The shorter players would hit him in the abdomen with their helmets. On one occasion, he tore his intestine and had to undergo abdominal surgery to repair the intestine. Also, there was the repeated concussion and broken bones. There was an ankle fracture as well.

Football success at Pacific Palisades High School came with a lot of football injury that I believe is part of the genesis of his substance use disorder. It is also important to note that during this time, his learning disability was slowly surfacing. He was dyslexic and had difficulty learning, which nobody knew at the time because he was doing well on the football field. The structure of football at high school was not as regimented as in the university, which he found out very quickly.

He was doing so well at Palisades High that he was appointed to give the class commencement address at graduation. I was very amazed at his articulation and how he got everyone laughing. All of the parents were proud of him, it seemed. If all these parents thought he was amazing, you can imagine what I felt as his mother. He had some big-name "friends" show up and were in the audience for him. He was happy that the school chose him and not the straight A student. It meant that they saw leadership in him as I did. When we thought of Jacques, we could never imagine substance use.

When he graduated from Palisades High and got a full scholarship to attend UCLA, he was happy. I was happy, and I felt he was on his way to do what he actually wanted to do. But UCLA didn't want him to play any other position other than a corner. They had recruited him to be a corner. When he got to UCLA, however, he decided that he wanted to play receiver. Apparently, he'd been watching Randy Moss and he felt that he could excel like Randy Moss as a player. He told UCLA that he wanted to play receiver, but to change a position like that, for which he was given a scholarship, was difficult. He had to sit out a lot because the receiver position was several players deep and they couldn't just push him right into receiver position. He had to wait.

At UCLA, Jacques's learning disability was becoming increasingly apparent. He had problems learning the playbook, especially as a receiver, a position he never played before. But neither me nor the university exactly knew that he had this learning disability because he was able to not display it very much. In the beginning when he wasn't playing like they needed him to play—such as following the theory of football—they thought that it was just because he was trying to be disobedient. But it was because he couldn't read the playbook, and this was a real problem throughout his time. When he wasn't getting a lot of playing time, he became more and more depressed.

The time at UCLA and the stress of being and unused talent caused Jacques deep pain, and he could not even communicate to anyone that he could not read the playbook. I believe this was the beginning of the substance use disorder. He also had a genetic predisposition to addiction because his paternal grandfather was depressed and an alcoholic.

Jacques did everything his friends told him to try. He tried to be buff and to be faster than his friends. He was experimenting with different substances. The senior students at UCLA gave him a lot of problems. There was a big hazing incident where he was hazed by an older student. Coming from the Church school, Jacques had never seen anything like that. He was very unhappy.

Now, this had come in light of the fact that my son had been sexually abused by his track coach, but he never shared it with anyone until years later. Jacques kept everything to himself and didn't know who to confide in. The track meet was out of town so the track coach said they had to go overnight to be there early in the morning for the track meet. Jacques was around fifteen at the time the abuse happened. This was something that he hid from me and from my husband. He carried all of these things in his chest, and these were all part of his problems. They're part of the genesis of his drug use. He started using steroids to build muscle. The pain of the sexual abuse, the pain of the failure to get a good film reel for pro tryouts, the pain of failed relationships . . . all of this was piling up and he felt lost. He dropped out of college after two years. Somehow, he managed to keep it together. Then like sunshine, a beautiful girl came along with God's gift, then two precious children. It was everything he ever asked for in life.

But underneath the surface, there was this disease that was slowly taking over in Jacques's brain. At first, he was occasionally using street drugs such as cigarettes, and marijuana. But as his depression and pain mounted, he used more drugs to fight the war in his head. His drug of choice was methamphetamine. He did not know how to provide for his family. He saw no way out, and he was believing a lie, that his wife could only continue to love him if he had a Lamborghini and a house like the one that he grew up in on the hill in the Palisades. All she wanted was a normal life with a partner who loved her.

But as a young man, it was difficult for Jacques to see the reality because everyone around him seemed to be living big lives. The professional football players had a lot of money and lived in big houses, and Jacques wanted to play professional football and believed he had the ability. No one doubted his ability, but he was not able to accept counsel from the people who could help him because he was using and putting things into his body that totally transformed the way he saw reality. In his warped reality, the substance was needed for survival in a world he believed was trying to suffocate him. But to the people looking at him and evaluating him, he appeared stubborn and unteachable. Yet nothing could be further from the truth. Even the pastor did not see his struggles. He would pray for him, but Jacques always went out and did again the very thing he had counseled him against.

By the time Jacques had his kids, he was not in the church. Yet the church is the place you need to be when you are newly married and have babies. That relationship was cut off. There was enough blame to go around. When you are not seeing correctly, it's everybody else's fault that things aren't going your way. When you are battling an illness like substance abuse, it's like your body is tied in a heavy chain and you're told to go swim. The support Jacques needed was at the church, as this was the foundation of strength, especially when you are ill. The people in the church might not understand, but they will eventually come around. You run to God, not away from God. His wife was willing and open to go to church with him even though she did not fully understand and never grew up in the church herself.

At the early phase when the children were young, Jacques was already out there deep in the drug scene. He had difficulty really focusing on the family. He was very distracted.

He was being fed street drugs. At one point, people would drive by on motorcycles and give him street drugs, such as cocaine. That was the beginning of the cocaine use. Now he had two drugs of choice: methamphetamine and cocaine. He did not understand the wedge that his change in character was driving between him and the woman that he fell in love with. He did not understand the damage that these drugs were doing to his body, especially his brain. What he thought was going to make him more appealing and stronger was actually driving a wedge between him and his loved ones and pushing them away. We did not fully know this new person. He would go for a week, and when he came back, he would get into arguments over the slightest issues. His feelings were sensitive and raw. His wife's position changed to the person protecting the children. The role of the father—this new character—was someone they did not know.

Now that we had established that my son had a substance use disorder (SUD), my great interest and time was spent in trying to find out more about this disorder. I wanted to know how it began and what caused it in my son. I could no longer close my eyes and wish that this nightmare would be gone when I woke up. I have come to learn that this is a disease, one that is chronic. It's not a tumor that you can cut out. This disease its unrelenting, and you manage it like you manage diabetes. You have to manage this chronic brain disease. A person can have a good quality of life and be productive if managed well. I went about first learning what my son was using and how he was getting it.

I learned that the substance use was self-medication by young people to treat their pain—the emotional pain and the physical pain. Whether it be from a football injury, a loss of a relationship, or a different part of rejection, these street drugs were readily available.

The oldest drug in America was the group of drugs called the *opiates* from the opium poppy seed. Since the 1940s, the source of the opium was from Mexico, and it was used to make morphine for the World War II efforts. After the war, the demand was cut down for legitimate use. The organized crime took over the market. There are different forms of the opiates: the brown tar, the white tar, and the black tar. The economics of the opiates have also changed with the arrival of synthetic opioids.

For example, heroin now includes other narcotics like fentanyl, OxyContin, oxycodone, and carfentanyl. Since 1957, opioids came and spread to America. By 1989, a typical heroin user was using Dilaudid and toluene, and mixed with tripelennamine. These patients and clients were seen in approved DEA clinics to dispense methadone. The clinics were very structured and well controlled.

It is believed that the first methadone clinic was established in Ohio. From Ohio, this clinic has proliferated to the rest of the country. For clarity, the use of methadone to treat heroin addiction was proposed by Dr. Marie Nyswander, a psychiatrist, and her husband, Dr. Vincent Dole, an endocrinologist. Both are now deceased. Their thinking was that methadone would be like diabetes where insulin, when injecting, could meet this physiologic need and demand of the organ and the body to regulate sugar. Then methadone could similarly be dispensed to meet the physiologic demands of the body by displacing the opioids on receptors and hence, be a controlled and non-habit-forming replacement for the body. As a result, remove the craving and addictive behavior pattern induced by the opioids and street heroin.

Nyswander and Dole tried this treatment method at clinics, and it worked, and many regular users of opioids were reporting that the cravings were reduced and some were gone totally. With this report in 1972, the FDA quickly approved methadone for the treatment of opioids disorder in the United States. The clinic mushroomed across United States. To this day, methadone is established as a gold-standard for heroin and opioid use disorder (OUD) of many kinds.

The result from the methadone clinic was phenomenal. Crime went down for users committing crime to feed their habits. Disease, such as hepatitis from sharing dirty needles, went down. HIV was better controlled. The users themselves were able to live a normal life, hold down jobs, pay taxes, and support their families. It was a win-win all around. Methadone clinics allowed management of drug use and allowed accurate data to be collected by the federal government about the extent of the problems in the US at large.

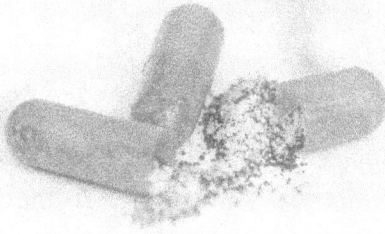

# Chapter 4

There was resistance in many states, especially the Ohio population, to methadone clinics. Many people died needlessly when they could have been enrolled in a methadone clinic. As times went by however, it became clear that the people in the methadone clinics were doing so well that at 60 to 65 milligrams every day of methadone, known as oral dosing, the euphoria from injecting heroin and opioids were blocked. *(SAMSHA, UNITED STATES)* Hence, people who were trying to get high by using other drugs while using methadone and heroin were just wasting their money. There was no gain, no euphoria, no high. No feel-awesome moment. They didn't experience anything but normal.

Methadone was very convenient in that it could be given once every twenty-four hours. The drug's half-life was long enough for the user to do a daily regimen and continue their lives. The methadone would be given orally, and it became the most oral drug used to treat any chronic substance use illness.

It is important to remember that methadone was not without its critics who argued that this opened the community to people they didn't really want to be in the community. As time went by however, it became clear that people in the methadone clinics were not just doing well, they were thriving. As the accumulated data became obvious, methadone would be the go-standard, not just in America, but in different parts of the world.

Once the methadone displaced the opioid and bonded to the primary receptor, the synaptic junction carrying the acylethanolamine was able to function normal. Thank God. The medically assisted treatment for opioid use disorder was now well established in the United States and comprehensive in all states of the union. Cognitive and Behavioral Treatment (CBT) was also combined with the medication-assisted treatment, and it has been found that individuals were able to live a fairly normal social life. With the cognitive treatment added to the methadone treatment, it became a very good comprehensive protocol for people with substance use disorder, especially opioid use disorder.

There are two major parts of the human being: the physical human, which you can feel and touch, and the spiritual human that you cannot see, which embodies most of life and allows life to be lived in the head and the heart.

We can be equally without understanding of the role this plays together to form the complete balanced person. We cannot be healthy without understanding the role that God plays and the spiritual part of our lives. The role of medicine is now finding ways to offer a comprehensive approach to care for people battling substance use disorder. It's not just giving them the cognitive treatment as well as the oral medication, but it's also to be able to offer therapy that involves spiritual healing as well.

In the early nineties, synthetic opioids flooded the market. The physicians were innocently prescribing medication and being used to dispense synthetic opioids like candies. Doctors were being bribed indirectly by aggressive marketing ploys designed by the pharmaceutical agents to prescribe synthetic OxyContin and oxycodone to patients who could have done just as good with Tylenol for ordinary pain. Doctors were told that these drugs were not habit forming, though the pharmaceutical companies knew full well that they were. A simple pain or dental extraction can become the initiation into substance use disorder by a lot of young people.

As time went on, the doctors were sent on expensive vacations and camouflaged conferences in exotic locations. They were just writing the prescription for this synthetic opioid without realizing that they were part of the problem and not part of the solution. The pharmaceutical companies were complicit, and then the doctors, who were initially innocent, were being drawn into the opioid use disorder that was spreading around the country.

Since 2014, there were companies that brought a drug called fentanyl into the United States and sold it as better than OxyContin and not habit forming. Hence, these companies knowingly developed a drug that their internal research told them was addicting and ten times more potent than the street heroin and OxyContin and allowed the doctors to write this prescription for pain management, when they knew that most of the doctors were not trained in pharmacology and did not fully understand the physiologic outcome of something like fentanyl.

Many kids died and many families were needlessly destroyed. How much money can you pay for such evil to compensate for that? People left the office with a prescription for OxyContin after a minor surgery or a tooth extraction. Doctors would combine fentanyl in pain treatment for office procedures. Naturally, the people came back asking for more pain treatment, for more OxyContin, and then the fentanyl became more available on the streets. Because the fentanyl and OxyContin were more expensive, the Chinese market stepped in and created a cheaper alternative to the more expensive pharmaceutical industry version. The knockoff version of the fentanyl that could be found on the streets from overseas shipment was now everywhere. The street version is like "falling off the trees," my son would say to me. Even the regular prescription of pain medication people attempted to fill online was tainted with fentanyl.

What is fentanyl? Fentanyl is a synthetic opioid similar to the opiate that grew as plants. The synthetic opioids are all made from chemicals formulated by uneducated people who have no concept of what these things can do to the human mind and body, and it's all for the sake of money. You are innocent parents, and your kids are the rat labs, except many kids die of an overdose before they can even tell you about it. Lots of these children die the very first time they try these drugs. How is that okay? A simple outing to hang out with their friends become a death trap, and you are left with a hole in your heart and grief from which you cannot recover.

What is happening is that the people who are using street drugs for the cheaper price do not know the difference. They just are happy they are getting a smaller amount of drugs that gave them an even bigger high and a bigger euphoria. The dealers who were making a fortune shipped these drugs into the US by the truckload and or by plane even before the DEA caught on and the fentanyl was all over the place. The users were combining fentanyl with heroin, cocaine, methamphetamine or anything that they could combine. We know, or hope, that the dealers are not trying to kill their customer—that would be counterintuitive. The outcome is nonetheless the same. The kids, the young adults, and the adults are succumbing at exceptionally large numbers and coming back in body bags after a night out of drugs and sex and what they think is fun. A casual evening of fun was resulting in death. Kids were overdosing, and parents were getting calls to come and identify their children or their family members in the morgues. While we know that the fentanyl is bad by the body count, there are many deaths that are not even reported. The dealers and the overseas street drug makers came up with an even stronger opioid by the name of carfentanyl. Carfentanyl is 10,000 times more addicting. This is a horse tranquilizer. A person who uses carfentanyl once will die.

In 2020, from physicians' data that was collected on drug-related deaths, the US government said there were about

100,000 deaths, but in reality, it is probably double that. In 2021, the reported deaths from fentanyl were about twice that. That's almost, 200,000 dead bodies.

The parents of Americans send their kids to great universities and to cope with the pressure of their young lives, to excel and to succeed, the kids take Adderall, called the "study pill." Adderall is huge on American college campuses and around the world. When combined with alcohol and fentanyl-laced Adderall, the crisis is huge.

Parents, let no one fool you, you must intervene in the lives of your kids. The evil forces that are out there to destroy their lives are more than you know, and it's massive. The federal government is doing everything they can to help the people at large, however, the policing of your kids, teenagers, and young adults is still your responsibility.

I'm writing this book to help you become more informed. There was a lot I did not know, especially as an immigrant mother and a professional person. Most of my life's work is taking care of people. Wake up, parents of America. If your kids have too much time on their hands and you can't control them, encourage them to go into the military. At least your chances of seeing them alive is higher. And if they do die, they will die for honor and something meaningful, like the service to their country and to their fellow man.

Nevertheless, it never crossed my mind in my wildest dream that I would send my son to an elite local university and there he would learn that if he took something from the street, it would give him the level of feel-good. He went to a parochial church academy and then onto public school before going to a big football university. Like most of you, even when my then daughter-in-law revealed to me what was going on, I played it down. I didn't fully know that the events of that day, when my grandkids did not come over, but it was God's way of showing me that danger was all around me. Thank God for prayer.

I took everything to prayer. I learned to pray very early. I remembered as a teenager my conversation with my dad. He said, "I want you to remember there are more problems resolved in prayer than this world knows." I wish now that I had fully understood the impact of those words at that time. I went on to make some choices that I would not have made today, but I thank God for those words and I learned to pray. I would pray sometimes five times a day, and my spirit became stronger for it. I continued to seek God fervently, and I understood the power of God.

I trusted the Lord that regardless of my error, or lack of knowledge, or ignorance in this area of addiction that the Lord Himself would provide for me and provide help for my kids. So when the workers of iniquity came against me, I was not afraid. The Lord has never let me down. He has been for me a mighty warrior.

The Lord told me, "Do not be afraid." Motorcycle gangs would drive by and hand my son cocaine. They put him in houses where drug dealers would drive by and hand them drugs in ODR Housing, and they made sure that the revolving doors to drug use were never closed. My son dug himself deeper and deeper into mental impairment and psychosis when he started using methamphetamines that they gave him, even for free. My son said to me, "Mom, these drugs are falling off trees like fruit. Everywhere I turn, someone is handing me drugs."

Methamphetamine and cocaine were my son's drugs of choice. These fit into the category called *stimulants*. Methamphetamine and similar drugs are known for their most destructive effects and damage to the body's organs. These drugs destroy the middle brain and the frontal cortex. And over time of use, methamphetamines and stimulants similar to it cause an increase in heart rate and blood pressure and can cause arrhythmias. An increase in blood pressure and heart rate has resulted in brain bleeds as seen in many autopsies of methamphetamine users.

The long-term users of methamphetamine have cognitive difficulties and will usually present to the emergency room repeatably with psychotic episodes or behavioral changes that cause legal issues. The users also have major sexual aggressive behavior causing problems and an increase in sexually transmitted diseases, such as HIV, as well as an increase in hepatitis and similar types of diseases where there's needle sharing. I thank God that my son managed to be protected from all these health problems by the power of the living God.

When people combine methamphetamine with cocaine or use cocaine occasionally with meth, they have a compounded effect and have severe cardiovascular damage. Cocaine exhibits severe toxicity to the heart muscle and heart valves. Methamphetamine will cause severe inflammation to the vessel. This inflammation will eventually lead to stiffness of the interior of the blood vessels and elevate blood pressure that causes the blood vessels, especially in the brain, to burst with pressure, resulting in bleeding in the brain, which is also known as a hemorrhagic stroke. People with opioid use will die from respiratory depression. What happens is the opioid and the heroin will make it difficult to breathe. So when someone on heroin combines it with fentanyl, knowingly or unknowingly, it depresses further the ability to breathe and they will eventually not wake up. It is recommended that family members and friends carry Narcan—a medication that reverses the symptoms of opioids—if they suspect a loved one is using any form of opioid or who has opioid use disorder. While people with opioid use disorder get help with methadone treatment and Suboxone treatment from many clinics around the country, people with stimulant use disorder do not have such treatment or such standardized programs. It is not clear why we are not more aggressive in finding ways to help these people, as damage to their health is more severe and they utilize the global health resource's more massively and are a greater burden for all taxpayers not just the parents.

It is important to note that at the time of this writing, no drug has been approved by the FDA for treatment of stimulant use disorder. Some drugs have been tried and tested and have shown promise, but nothing has been approved. Dr. Philip Coffin at the University of San Francisco, who is an expert in stimulant use disorder, has done some extensive studies about some drugs that show significant promise even in combination with other drugs that could be used to decrease the craving for methamphetamine, or maybe possibly decrease the death rate. But, again, nothing has been approved yet by the FDA.

Substance use disorder (SUD) in general is a serious health problem, one requiring a lot of resources. Lives lost cannot come back. This is America's potential. How can America compete with countries where 99 percent of their population has intact brain function? For both opioid use disorder and methamphetamine use disorder, we see loss to the communities in death of promising younger lives, loss to the families associated with pain, and holes left that nothing could fill. Families and friends are left with this loss and pain, these empty seats missing from the dining room table, and there seems to be nothing they can do.

But there is something we can all do, from the drug dealers to the preachers to the people using these drugs. The drug dealers' bosses can use their drug profit to make sure they take drugs off the streets that are killing people. Parents can make sure their kids don't leave the house when they don't know where they are going or who their friends are. Politicians can go to Washington, and instead of bickering and fighting all the time, they can pass legislations that will help people who are suffering from addiction have stress-free lives, letting everyone in America have a place they can call home and a community that cares about young people. Faith-based organizations can cooperate with the government to create meaningful programs that are sustained to strengthen American families.

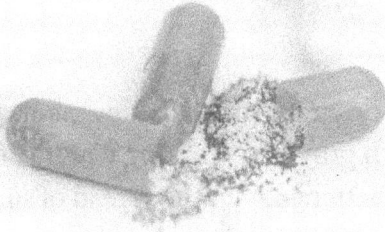

# Chapter 5

There is a mass incarceration problem in the United States related to drug use. The courts and legal system don't seem to know what to do with a large number of people within the legal system who have behavioral problems associated with drug use. The mass incarceration is causing the taxpayers more and more every year. Now that the prisons are privately run, there's no real incentive to find appropriate ways of treating these people outside of the prison system.

It has become evident that there needs to be a serious shift in the care of people with substance use disorder. The problem has become so severe that business as usual with the revolving door of imprisonment has not added any benefit. When there is massive proliferation of substance use that causes mass psychosis, cardiac disease, brain disease, multiorgan disease and multiorgan failure, and death, then lawmakers must be willing to commit significant funding to a comprehensive approach to the treatment of drug use disorder. A model treatment approach and facility will need to be included. Housing and social programs need to be part of this new program that provides medical treatment early enough with providers working with the families and communities to better contain the spread of substance use. It appears that the doctors who know the most about these problems are the ones with the least amount of support to help lead solutions to these problems.

The families and friends, community leaders, political leaders, worship leaders, and the pastors need to be integrated in the resources available to care for substance abuse users. It's particularly important that the faith-based organizations are included since there is a spiritual connection that we have seen with substance use disorder. It's important to include the churches, religious leaders, Christians, and Muslims, and the pastors in community. We need to make sure that the synagogues and the leaders of these communities are included in whatever care and program is being created. It should not be a profit-making entity when this type of problem exists in the community that is destroying the very fabric of society. Profit should not be the driver in these programs. There should be enough to be paid a living wage but not hoarding money at the expense of people with real problems. The truth is that people who do not see or believe in the urgency of finding solutions to these problems will not be able to enjoy their own lives with time. Parents are being gauged by these revolving-door rehabilitation facilities that offer nothing but bandages to serious open wounds. There is little incentive to really help people recover.

The drug problem in America is everybody's problem. It is a disease, and the people who suffer from substance use disorder are not able to help themselves. If we left diabetic individuals without serious medical programs, community, and individual education, we would not have the control we have in diabetes care. This problem is not just an individual problem—this is a national problem and a global problem.

Every country in the world has adopted the diabetes treatment program. Similarly, a global approach needs to be taken in the care of people with substance use disorder because it's everywhere. It's a very massive problem. The support of the federal government, the pharmaceutical industry, the private endowments, the university programs and alike all need to come together in creating a sustainable treatment program that can help people with substance use disorder, not just in America, but all over the world.

How many more kids and young people need to die before this problem becomes a problem that people really show great interest in? This is not a problem of poor people. This is not a problem of people "over there." This is a problem of everyone. This is a problem that knows no zip code. This problem is in the boardrooms of America, in universities, in grade schools. This problem is in homes and affects everyone, from the soccer mom to the firefighters. This is a problem that's everywhere. Hence, we all must come together to create a program and a comprehensive way to treat people with all form of substance use disorder, not just opioid disorder with methadone and Suboxone (treatment for opioid addiction), but also for people with the stimulant use disorder, especially in the face of fentanyl contaminating everything.

I have learned a lot from my son and the battle to save his life. I learned a lot about brain disease and how substance abuse users are marginated and have been used as a racquet for unscrupulous money-making programs, enriching people who do not care for your children. The insurance companies are not providing blanket or broad enough care to be able to make this affordable for the families who are dealing with this difficulty. The rehabilitation programs—a pathetic house of horror with revolving-door facilities—take advantage of families in crisis. They do not want to accept what insurance pays, which is not much, so families are forced to borrow money or mortgage their home to pay for their loved one to stay at the facility. Usually a stay is thirty days, sixty days, or maybe a little bit more, and then the funds run out and the loved one is released back onto the street where the cycle of abuse will continue.

It is important that everyone comes together to face this issue head-on. Government grants should be given for providers who are willing to head these meaningful programs that is not bogged down in bureaucracy. We must elect officials who are interested in really helping substance users, helping families receive proper care, and will help stop the widespread availability of these drugs in the community. You don't need to be a medical doctor with a son in crisis to care about the health and wellbeing of substance users and to want to change the shameful system. People seem to find money to do just about anything that they want, but our greatest resources is the investment in human beings, an investment in our people, and those in need are getting the least amount of care.

Substance use disorder is a serious health problem. When users are not on the street, they are shackled in chains and behind bars, which makes money for the private prison's merchants. The crisis is such that if we don't pay attention and shift the blame to someone else, then we will all suffer from this problem. There is not enough manpower for law enforcement to help curb this problem. The criminal activities around drug sales and use and the illegal manufacturing is too much for law enforcement to handle it alone. The victim with substance abuse carries all the burden of punishment and suffering while the private companies run to the bank with the money.

The time has come when we must all step up. The large infrastructure bill that is pending signature by President Biden must dedicate a large sum to combat this disease with infrastructure of smart rehabilitation facilities, rehabilitation buildings, and education for families and people with this disease. Allocating funds for prevention programs, starting from the home, the school, and the universities. The small rehab facilities that use mental problems and substance abuse as a meal ticket need to stop. Human suffering cannot be a money-making entity in this way when most of the time the outcome is death.

Most families in the United States are unable to put their kids into programs that can protect them from getting into drugs. Some families are headed by single parents, fathers, or mothers who are not able to be at home to watch their children all the time or have nannies to help at critical ages to help parents. There should be places where parents and children can get the care, training, and the education they need to understand what these drugs can do to their bodies and their health early enough when they can avoid these problems.

If there was funding for faith-based organizations—church, synagogues, and mosques—then families could get the support and training that they need. So we need to pull in great men of God, like Evangelist Franklin Graham, Pastor Harold Warner, Rob Scribner, Pastor T.D. Jakes, Pastor Joel Osteen, Pastor T. Shuttleworth, Pastor Rudy Hagood, Pastor Rick Warren, Pastor Isaiah Saldivar, Bishop Charles Blake, Bishop Kenneth Ulmer, Joyce Meyer, Steve Furtick, and other religious leaders from the Muslim community, like Imam Omar of the Ricky Islamic Center of Southern California. Additionally, Rabbi Lauren Holtzblatt from the Adas Israeli synagogue, and Rabbi Steven Z. Leder from Wilshire Boulevard Temple Synagogue. These organizations see many kids and families when the kids are young. The government should partner with these organizations at the grassroot and not keep creating programs that do not work.

Kris Jenner has managed to raise six well-grounded kids who are not on drugs. One of her beautiful daughters became the youngest billionaire in America. The greatest thing is that they know Jesus Christ. Her daughter Kim Kardashian is so talented and smart and has many young followers. She funded the 90 Day to Freedom campaign that helps nonviolent drug offenders get released from prison. Kim's ex-husband, mogul Kanye West, has many young followers as well, so instead of the kids going to steal to buy the shoes, maybe Kanye can help these kids have a drug-free life and teach them that his shoes look better when you are not on drugs.

It is critical that these type of grounded people and institutions that hold communities and the American system together be involved in the solution to substance use disorder. The COVID-19 pandemic is in the frontline and COVID is everywhere, but nobody seems to be saying very much about substance use disorder in the face of COVID or made worse by COVID. Yet over 200,000 kids die yearly from this wicked drug, especially when combined with alcohol. People came together quickly to battle COVID, with research, science, etc., why can't they do that with substance abuse?

We have observed that the disease of substance use has a significant spiritual element associated with it. So it's become more important that we include faith-based organizations in permanent solutions, as opposed to just warehousing people, incarcerating them as punishment, as this does not really change the outcome over time. How many more kids need to die before it becomes something that everybody is interested in?

I am solidly Christian in my affiliation, but I am not ignorant to think that this is just what one particular group of people can handle. This problem requires the input of every person to be able to handle and curb the spread of substance use in America and in the world at large.

This is not a political matter. This is a battlefield for the soul of America. I am pleading with the current administration, President Biden and Dr. Jill Biden, to please put together a committee and a program that can help find solutions to this problem, as if it were a war we are fighting. I'm asking you to please ask Congress and the Senate to appropriate funding specifically for substance use disorder, especially to faith-based organizations to be able to help out in creating a sustained program where the children are taught early, before anybody even pressures them into any substance use that these things are completely not right for their body.

The Band-Aid treatment does not work. It does not work in America. And we see that this is what America currently offers its kids: Band-Aid treatments that do not work on a very serious disease. America is the greatest country in the world.

For most families, from what we have seen, from data collected by CDC and many respected government and private institutions, substance use disorder can start as early as eight years old when the children and families do not even fully know what's going on, especially when the children's brains are just being formed and they're using substances that affect their frontal cortex and their cognitive ability. This is a destruction that follows them through life.

The dumbing down of America. It appears that the American model is that when we have not supported our people and our kids to be strong emotionally and cognitively, and mothers and fathers have to work to support their families. We just warehouse the kids with substance abuse issues in prisons and bring in people from other countries that can fulfill the labor requirements in the U.S. Very shameful. Isn't America supposed to lead the world to good? While they are in prison they should be trained and gain the skills needed for reentry back into society.

The kids in grade schools, and from their interaction with other children, are expressing unhappiness in school and with their peer groups. Their social interaction becomes problematic. They are feeling isolated and depressed. This is a period when children need activity that stimulates the happy brain section of the cortex. They do not need to be put on drugs. They need to be in environments that encourage them and teach them early that God is very present with us wherever we are.

Children love adult and peer interaction where everyone is affirmed. Children who watch a lot of TV early in life and play video games do not develop strong survival social skills, rather, they have a strong, aggressive spirit that is self-focused. We know that kids who are in single family homes or broken homes may not have a lot of resources. Hence, we build smart cities where these very programs are teaching children that the world belongs to God, we are here on a journey to eternity.

The children who are highly active do not need ADHD drugs at such an early age. They do not need to put kids on medication for every little sign of sadness. Can a safety net be placed around the young kids to enjoy the outdoors and get to know and help each other? Do kids need opioids or pain control when they go in for simple dental work? This casual use of wrong treatment for minor pain and discomfort is laying the foundation for substance use disorder. There is familiar connection with substance use disorder and depression. Families with depression appear to show a predisposition to substance use disorder. As a result, these kids and families need special selection of treatment that does not drive them into drug-seeking behaviors.

Healthy and positive activities, food, and social interaction and reinforcement is important early in life. In high school, when teens are more interested in peer interaction, we need to provide an environment where they can develop non-self-focus but develop good self-image and not isolation.

Children need to understand a life of service to fellow human beings early on in their development. Even when there is some degree of mental illness, children who have learned to serve even their own sibling tend to do better in life, in general.

Everything should be done to encourage the fathers to engage with their children early in life. When men are not gainfully employed and have free-flowing use of alcohol, marijuana, and pornography, the very fiber of the family and children's lives is disrupted. We all have free choices, but substances like alcohol, tobacco, and drugs readily available becomes a problem for people who are predisposed to this brain disease. Sports injury in young kids has also played into this brain disease. We now know that early concussion in high school teenagers or grade school children presents major learning problems. We also know that childhood traumas, whether emotional or physical, are related to disease development. Early loss of emotional care and support is very devastating in the adult coping mechanism. These young people develop depression, substance use disorder, and various diseases, also childhood sexual abuse, which is so pervasive in our world, it is destructive to our children and our society at large.

Sexual abuse is believed to play a strong role in substance use disorder in America. There is deep pain associated with sexual abuse in young children as they try to mask this pain with drugs and self-medication. When people feel deep pain, especially emotional pain, we know that no amount of medication works, but the quick, temporary euphoria for opioids and stimulants provides a temporary escape from a state of no-way-out, as these young people believe they are trapped in deep, emotional trauma. They can only be healed by the truth of God's word. Jesus said to his disciples, "It is the Spirit who gives life; the flesh profits nothing; the words that I speak to you are spirit, and they are life." (John 6:63, NKJV). Why are parents not giving their kids this gift of life? Rather, what we see is the work of the flesh leading to death all around us.

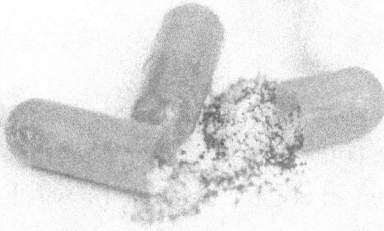

# Chapter 6

What I learned from my son has been very useful about this disease, and I feel obligated to share with other parents and families why it is important to know early about this disease. If you know early on what your kids are going through, you can help steer them to a solution that will help their problems. You can seek professional help for them early. Their sense of isolation in dealing with what is going on in their head is then discussed in the family and they know they do not have to suffer alone. You can help them manage peer pressure. I learned that they feel really depressed after things don't turn out the way they expected in their lives. These kids feel pain, perhaps even deeper than adults.

I learned that the hazing in football programs is destructive to many people and should not be encouraged. I learned that fights in locker rooms or the bullying leads to a sense of isolation and despair, and it becomes a health issue and a pain issue for those who are being bullied. My son came from a Christian home and was not familiar with the things he was seeing and experiencing at school, and he began to feel ashamed and attacked. There was also the incident with the track coach who abused him. He said he felt very depressed in college because he was having problems understanding the academic playbook, he became more depressed and isolated. At the time, I was busy finishing school and confident that my son was already in his dream program at a big university. I focused on my work, and he lived on campus, and for months I never saw him. When I did see him, it was brief and nice, and everything went back to normal life.

Even though a lot of people were around him, my son was trying to fit in and he was living life alone. There was name-calling and the pressure to fit in. He's thin-built and fine-faced and was picked on. So his friends in the senior class told him that he could buff up with steroids and growth hormones so he could be stronger and run faster. He began to try these things. He was given limited play time because he had changed the position on the football team. He was brought into the UCLA football program to play the corner position, but he wanted to play a receiver. He believed that he was better built for receiver. This was a critical mistake for him because he had to wait for a receiver position to open up.

It also meant he had to be moved away from the coach who recruited him and move to a different coach who did not know him very well except from film reels as a running back to which he won All Star and All-American Awards. All these serious life changes were going on, and there was no father to guide him through. I don't know much about football and neither did his stepfather. His stepfather grew up working on a strawberry farm in Bellingham, Washington, and never threw a ball in his life. Because of the abuse from his friends when he was not getting much play time, Jacques decided to change schools to a smaller football program in San Diego. At this point, I was wondering why he wanted to leave such a storied program to go to a lesser known one away from his home and a city that had followed him in the newspapers from high school.

I knew it was the wrong move, and I did all I could do to discourage it. He was sinking more into depression and unhappiness. In San Diego, he went straight in as a receiver with a great coach. The receiver lineup was deep, and he had to sit out a year following NAAC rules. He eventually got some playing time, but it was few and far between. Knowing his time to play college football was running out, he decided to return back to the big university program he left in UCLA. They welcomed him back, but he had to sit out another year based on NAAC rules, and the clock was ticking to get playing time as a receiver.

My son's academics suffered. Knowing he was suffering, and it was visible now, I did not want to push academics or make him stay and finish his degree. He dropped out of UCLA and started trying out for professional football anyway as well as a private receiver anywhere. He enrolled with a private receiver coach to receive one on one coaching. Like with every great receiver, my son traveled where the great receivers were, he wanted to go and I paid for whatever they said the cost was, but the depression and pain was such that when we arrived at this program, Jacques refused to participate as requested of him, and the coach did not think he was playing full out or giving his best. Cris Carter was especially eager to help him, but Jacques had lost motivation and it seemed that the fight was no longer in him. We went to as many football combines as possible, from state to state, but he did not get the call back.

Jacques sunk into more depression without knowing it, but about this time he began to use substances to treat pain and cope with rejection. Then there were his earlier football injuries from broken bones to the intestinal tear and concussion. Everything was now coming together to create this load of pain and burden he was carrying by himself. His biological father was irresponsible and was never available to help him, so my son cried for his father who never showed up and for the stepfather unable to help. He was afraid of financial responsibility of a son that was not his, a task I never asked for myself. I was happy doing my normal work and being a wife and a mother to the boys. I was in solo practice and made myself available to drive them wherever they needed to go for sports.

When my son was told not to return to the church, because he was involved with the associate pastor's daughter without approval, it was heartbreaking all around. Then he met another beautiful girl from Canada. The whole situation was so dramatic. In his young life, he had lived a life that most people never lived their entire life. He was well traveled and involved in missionary work. At this point, he had advanced to methamphetamine use. I was traveling and trying to figure out ways to make a living outside of the local area. During this time, he met and married his beautiful wife. When I first saw her, she was already expecting their first child. I loved her immediately. To this day, it is not clear if she knew how I cared for her. As ravages of substance use was already playing out in my son, slowly at first, he kept it together and they had some fun times and were very much in love. Then the baby came and shortly after, their second child. The question was how he could provide for his family. The level of depression had now risen to a high level, and he was not being treated, except by his use of street drugs. His young wife was nevertheless devastated. She didn't know how to help him. He was beginning to lash out at the very people he loved so much, and their lives daily were difficult.

His emotions were very raw. If you even looked at him cross-eyed, he was ready to pick a fight, and throw and move the tables around. He would go a few days at a time and say nothing to his wife. On several such days, he would stop by my house in Santa Monica after not having talked to his wife for days. His wife's family began to see that he was not happy. When under the drug influence, he would flirt with his wife's friends and even offer them substance. It eventually got back to his wife that he was hitting on her friends; this was most distressing to his young wife, and she was unhappy.

On a beautiful spring morning in Santa Monica, California, I was waiting for my daughter-in-law to bring over my two grandkids, as she normally did every day. I babysat the children three days a week, and they saw their other grandmother on the other days. When they had not shown up and no one had called me, I called my daughter-in-law. In a serious voice and tone, which I had never heard from her before, she told me she would not be bringing the kids over. She said that my son—her husband—had used street drugs in the backyard of their house. This information hit me like a ton of bricks. My first thought was that she was upset about his coming and going, but I didn't want to believe that he was using street drugs, and certainly wasn't bringing drugs to their house.

I always felt that I taught my boys well and they were God-fearing people. Our lives were built around the word of God, church, family, and work. So I prayed for God's help and for clarity. From that day forward, I was determined to try to understand what was going on and that I would hold no judgment until I had talked to my son. To put things into perspective, this was during the 2008 housing crisis, and I was in the danger of losing my beautiful home in Santa Monica, California. My income was greatly slashed. My doctor's practice was floundering, and the years of great success as a sole physician practitioner was seriously compromised.

As l battled to save my home and my practice, the time with my grandkids, who were ages 1 and 3 at the time, was my greatest source of comfort. They were born healthy and beautiful, and I was a great part of their care for at least three days of the week. I looked forward to the time I spent with them. We would walk to the park or I would carry them in a buggy. They were happy and thriving. We would go to the library and check out books, or I would read the books there. This went on for about a year and we were all happy. I looked forward to the time that I was with them regularly. In the evening, my daughter-in-law would pick the children up when she got off work. All that was missing at the time was finding ways to get my business going again. At one point when I was out of town, my son and his family lived in my house. The children had gotten to know my house as their home in Santa Monica. After I returned from Texas, I watched and I noticed that my son was anxious and unhappy, and he appeared depressed. He was hypersensitive to everything. His conversations with me were mainly about how he would provide for his family. He was thirty-three at the time. They moved to an apartment in Venice, California, and I would go over there and babysit to help them. My daughter-in-law also appeared quite unsettled and unhappy.

One year, I was invited to spend Thanksgiving with my daughter-in-law's family. She came from a large family, and I wanted to get to know them better. Thanksgiving was being hosted at her father's house near San Diego. There were nine kids—three girls and six boys—and that was eleven family members with the parents. It reminded me of my family. When my son was a baby, he had gone to Africa and lived with my large family for about 4 years. My daughter-in-law came from a great family. Her mother was very motherly, and it appeared that she really enjoyed the role of motherhood. She and her husband were separated. I thought my daughters-in-law father was friendly and engaging, a good gentleman. Her mother cooked and she baked. She was very present. She still had the element of a German European in her. The family owned a furniture business, and the dad mainly ran that business. Thanksgiving was well, no drama, and everyone was happy and welcoming. For the first time, I got to meet and really become familiar with all the people and a few of the friends of the family. I thought to myself at the time, this is a lovely family, to whom my son had correctly married in. One of the sons went to school with my son in Pacific Palisades High School. I felt my son was okay and if he did well with his sport and finished school, he would have a great family of his own.

As time went on, it became increasingly clear to me that my son had substance use problems. I noticed him leaving for a week at a time before he would return, he would sleep for hours and he often looked disheveled. I began to slowly understand the impact of this reality, and I paid greater attention to everything. I was concerned about the children, and I wanted them to never feel neglected. I tried to make our time together count. I would ask him what was going on and he admitted that he was taking a substance for body building.

I would video document my time with the children as I saw that they were really having fun, and I wanted them to remember when they were grown that their childhood was very happy. I always wished I had ways of seeing myself when I was younger. I also documented the time when my son was with the children and how he interacted with them. When their mother picked up the children, I would video document how she was looking and how her mood was. I'm sure she saw me videotaping, but it wasn't until recently that I realized the important value of these video recordings.

My grandchildren's interest was one of my greatest concerns. They were my first grandchildren, and I wanted to help them understand that no matter what was going on, I wanted them to be happy. I wanted their childhood to be as much fun and creative as possible. Whether they were around me or anyone else, I wanted their childhood to be memorable. Little did I know that this video documentation would bring great clarity for my son and my daughter-in-law's life at a different time in their lives. Drug use had come into their lives and also my life. It was leaving a mark of pain, loss, regret, and brokenness. There were a lot of unknowns and anxiety as I watched them. The Lord gave me the peace that whatever happened I could trust Him.

Eventually his wife got a job to support herself and the kids as a designer. She was so good at her job and was making good income, so her family began to advise her to dump him.

His wife was close to big media and celebrities, so everyone came to her rescue while my son was isolated and depressed. People told her that that he should not be involved in their lives, their photographs, and not in the lives of her kids, and that she shouldn't be around him. It's important to note that the life my son knew growing up had been fairly without lack of anything he wanted. He lived in a big house with views of the Pacific Ocean for eleven years of his life, and then we moved to Santa Monica in a smaller house. With a divorce from his stepfather, my son understood the importance of supporting his family, and this was a major stress factor as well for him.

His stepfather had spent over twenty years building a skin-care business. The business was good for us, and we were able to live the American dream. In addition to the medical practice, our business supplied products to doctors around the US who were doing well. Then came 9/11 and the Patriot Act, and someone targeted me and ran me out of business. Our main source of income was suddenly gone. My patients would be canceling appointments. I never worked for anyone, so it was hard to cope and transition to a nine-to-five job. My sons, who were being groomed to take over the business for their families, suddenly had nothing to step up on. The football was not there, and all attempts to rebuild the product business for my son's young family was limited because there was nowhere to set up the production company. Let's just say that this was a crisis.

My son tried to sell his paintings, but without knowledge or marketing, which did not convert. So he was a struggling artist. When he would be high on methamphetamine and get upset at every little thing, he thought everyone was trying to put him down, so he began to push away his very source of healing— his family and source of comfort—because he could not provide for them. He took odd jobs, such as delivering furniture. There was no way out of the methamphetamine obstacle. The drug damaged the frontal cortex area of his brain, as well as the middle brain region. The disease had now progressed. The behavioral problem was associated with low morals, low self-esteem, focused on sexual activity, poor cognitive function, poor empathy, and everything was switched backwards. The people who were vulnerable—his kids and wife—were not being cared for. The wife's family, especially her brothers who had their own issues, were now picking fights with my son and calling him names.

In one such situation, there was a verbal back and forth and I was on the line trying to calm the one brother down. It was very clear to me that they were already too upset and there was nothing I could say that would make them feel any better. That gave me a little opening as to where we were and how bad things had gotten. I prayed for them, and I believed that the hand of the law had protected my daughter-in-law and the babies. It was clear in my heart that she really loved him, and I know he loved her. So knowing that the Lord can do all things, even though she was not a believer that the Lord would help her while my son tried to find himself. She moved with her kids to be with her family.

I decided to focus on service to the poor and rebuild a non-profit organization, Doctors and Nurses to the World International Foundation, I created in 1994 as Lighthouse Doctors and Nurses International, at the same time figuring a way to help my son survive and be there for his kids. I know no matter how good people are, they will never be a father to my son's kids. These kids know they have a dad, and I can just imagine the pain of loss they must have felt when their dad suddenly stopped showing up. Fathers are very important in the lives of their children, and when America finds a way to support and encourage men to be real dads, to be real partners and not all sexually focused, then the children of America would be stronger and do much better.

I lost my home in Santa Monica, which was yet another upheaval for my son. The place he would show up to and lay out was now gone.

My second son also took this extremely hard. The loss of the home that he had mostly grown-up in. He went to live with his father after the divorce, then he moved out and got himself a studio apartment which was only a place that he lived by himself. My second son did not have a place to move to after we lost the home. However, the kids were no longer kids; they were men and had not found their way. They needed their dad, but he was not there for them. We were dealing with disruption of the fabric of our lives and did not know where to turn.

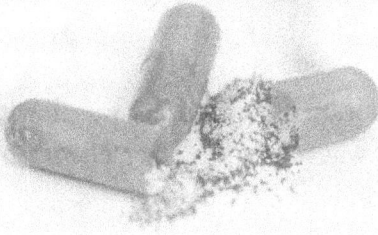

# Chapter 7

My son said that his drug use was mainly one gram of methamphetamine daily. He was manifesting body dysmorphia and disliked his looks and himself. He started wearing large round earrings and getting tattoos. He tattooed his face and would gather things on the street he found in dumpsters. He would try to bring these things to his wife, but she wanted none of it. This was before the COVID-19 pandemic. He would show up at all times of the night and try to leave furniture or the things he'd picked up for her. Even the neighbors would be upset and would sometimes call law enforcement.

He was now living on the street for several days at a time. He was losing all concept of his normal family life. At one point, he lived with his grandmother (my mother). He would use methamphetamine and would go to his grandmother's house to stay for weeks until he got the craving to use again. The cycle was repeating for months and years. He barely saw his family and kids, and I was very far away in China. He would often take long walks wearing poor clothing and barely any shoes. This was very bad, and his health was deteriorating. My mother was ill with end-stage lung disease and was incredibly stressed watching her first grandson deteriorate.

When Jacques was a year and a half old, he went to live with my parents and spent about five years in Nigeria. When I finished my medical training and internship, he returned back to United States. By then, I had moved to Los Angeles, California, doing my postgraduate work. I was overjoyed to be reunited with my son. He was amazing and beautiful. To make the transition easier for him, my mother came back with him.

He had his mom and his grandmother, but his dad was never there. My dad and brother were the men in his life earlier. They supported him. He was very happy. The house in Nigeria was full of people who just loved him. They would drive him around and he would play with all the kids his age. There was plenty of ice cream. My parents were wholesalers for frozen food for the area and were well-known. They supplied frozen food to the university, to the market, and the hotels.

Jacques was happy in Africa. He was the American baby who came to live with his grandparents' family. He had crowds of the kids around him that he played with. Returning to America, Los Angeles was a culture shock for him. He missed his friends. He missed my dad, his grandpa. He missed his nanny and all the bicycle boys who came to distribute ice cream on bikes and had made sure he had any flavor he wanted.

Soon after arriving in Los Angeles, I tried to enroll him at the SEED school. He also attended the summer kids' sports camp at the university in Westwood. But it was clear that he was not in his element. Everything was too structured. He missed the African outdoors and freedom.

Soon thereafter, I met my then husband and after a year, we decided to get married and provide a most stable home for my son. I was in dermatology clinical research fellowship and doing low-income jobs. Our marriage was beautiful. First, the engagement at the Beverly Hills Hotel with my research associates and every one of the doctors I had come to know there. It was beautiful. Followed with a wedding months later at the university church in Westwood. And the wedding reception at the Riviera Country Club . . . everything was perfect. I felt like a princess.

We bought a three-bedroom house in the Mar Vista area and had our little place to begin our marriage. I was working as hard as I could. My family stayed over up to the wedding. They soon moved in with us. This is the African way, where the first kid essentially was responsible to help take care of the family.

My husband, from a small town, lost both parents very early in life. His upbringing was totally different. He had two brothers. And these men essentially readied themselves with occasional help from their grandmother and aunts. Their parents left a forty-acre farm for the boy. My husband grew up working in a strawberry farm to support himself. His whole life had been about taking care of himself.

When he married me, he now had to be father to a six-year-old boy who was very hungry to have a father he did not have. He did not know how to do it. He also did not know how to handle my family that were now living with us. There was also job insecurity for him in the early part of our marriage. He was not able to cope with everything. The marriage began to strain, but for ten years we kept it together.

We had my second son. He came out with his eyes wide open, ready to conquer the world. He was a good, strong child. And I knew at the time that he had the potential to go as high as he wanted to go. We moved into a large house in Pacific Palisades, California. The kids were happy in the Palisades.

Our older son played football. He did not want to play in Church Academy football. He wanted to play in a bigger school. He excelled academically and in sports. He was not a straight A student. But he did well enough to stay on the football team. He became the star and got the attention he never got at the smaller Church Academy.

At the church school there were mostly lovely families. They were clicked in commitment to the Bible reading. The pastor himself, a former football player, ran a tight ship. He really tried to help my son when he saw that he needed a father and a guardian. He even had him move into his own house to thrive in that environment when he was about sixteen.

When you had poor structure and an absent father, you will not do well. Very few young men with absent fathers early in life did well in an environment like that. Some of the boys got into marijuana use and smoking and sex earlier than they needed to be in their teenage years. The pastors were not having it. And I agreed with him.

I always had great respect for the pastor and his family. A Black woman with a big degree was a fish out of water in Santa Monica, California. We went on two medical missions to West Africa and South America. I had organized to start the church's medical mission to Sierra Leone. I was pleasantly surprised that the book written by the church, which was put together by the assistant pastor and the other physician in the church, and the pediatrician, gave me credit for leading the first medical mission to West Africa. That was very surprising. I did not expect that at all. That was respectable.

When people targeted me, the assistant pastor's wife, elder and schoolteacher, along with her precious dad, Poppy, (I will never forget get him), stood in prayer for me. For one year the pastor's wife would pray with me at 6:00 a.m. prayer and encouraged me to trust God, knowing that his grace is sufficient in every situation. With my own eyes, I saw how the Lord fought for me.

Now fully immersed in the drug culture, my son began to change his looks to fit the drug life. The earrings and the tattoos got more pervasive. Wherever there was space in his body, he tattooed. When his brother made the mistake of buying him a home tattoo kit to try to correct a bad tattoo job, he had no idea that he'd opened a can of worms. My son tattooed everything, including his eyeballs, to make him look the part of the movie hero he loved. It was now self-destruction.

The methamphetamine has driven him into temporary psychosis. He had no idea how bad things had gotten for him. When he stopped using and agreed to go into rehab, in 2015 - 2016 he cleaned up. He even found himself a church near his grandmother's house and was near enough that he could walk to the church on Sundays.

When he did not use meth, my son was functioning well, and he was accepted into the church choir. He would sing with the choir, and he worked at the church for about a year, building a new church relationship. One of the junior pastors who had a past history similar with substance use disorder was very welcoming to my son. But when Jacques saw the kids at church and the fathers with their kids, he would get the trigger of pain. That pushed him to relapse time and time again. All the wonderful gains he had made went out of the door. Yes, his children's absence was a pretty bad trigger, and every time he would think about them, he would relapse. Once he used, he felt better. This pattern of drug use was very consistent. Something usually around his ex-wife would trigger his sadness and sense of loss and he would take off. He was most sad that he let her and the kids down and did not know how to heal that. A few times he had attempted to kill himself to release her of any more pain.

He said his grandmother was a rock for him. She was always there when he was a baby. Then one morning while I was still in London, I received the telephone call that I dreaded my whole life. It was my sister in the UK calling to tell me that my mother had passed away. That was about as hard as anything could have been for me. I screamed. I cried and cried. It was such a painful call. It was like the whole world wanted to steal from me. As a physician, I had spent years trying to figure out how to help my mother heal her dying lung. No one knew or understood my suffering. Losing my mother to this illness was really hard for me. It was not something I could fix.

The stem cell research that I was beginning to understand was not readily available in the United States at that time. If you wanted it, you had to go to a place like Ukraine. Ukraine hospitals were claiming 75 percent success in recruiting the lung cells. It would not have been easy to get her there because of the twenty-four hours of oxygen that she was using.

Jacques could have helped me with her, but he was not doing well. I could not even discuss my pain with anyone, not even members of my own family, because they had no idea of my suffering, and they were forming the opinion that I was not there. My younger sister and brothers were already having disagreements about how one of my brothers took away my children's inheritance, my children's future, with my company that I worked so hard to build over twenty years. They somehow could not get themselves to understand, that I worked so hard to build and to help all of us. That income from my company was important for me and my children.

It took me twenty years to build the company, and $25,000 is not what a professional person gets after the effort. Whatever the case, I prayed for the Lord to help me to overcome, to forgive, and to help me to try to move on. Then there was the condominium that I had purchased for my mother. I did not write any will or contract that stated if anything happened to my mother that the property needed to come back to me and my children, and then they could buy them out or give them back any interest they might have. I just assumed that we were all family and were working toward the common goal to strengthen our family. But that was not what happened. Me and my children were left in the cold. Everything was lost. My grandchildren got nothing. So one of my brothers took from me, even though I was the one who was instrumental in feeding him for years. But nonetheless, it was the Lord that fed all of us, and because the Lord fed us, one cannot go back to yesterday. My mother is now dead. I was not able to help her. Now, all of my three homes—the Victorian house in Buffalo, the big house in Santa Monica, and the condominium—are gone. All my resources were taken from my children. So my sons found themselves without the inheritance they thought would come to them. They all had to start over.

After my mother's passing, I returned to the United States. My mother looked like an angel. In my eyes she was. I couldn't say anything wrong that she ever did to me. I wanted to be holding her hands when she passed away, the pain was deep. The pain of seeing her and my sons suffer was very deep. The disappointment my second son felt in the loss of our home was deep. It seemed that I was very good at giving away everything to everyone but never had protected myself or my children.

Why didn't I give thought to the possibly to that which was built with so much sweat and suffering, a Black woman at my level of success as an immigrant who lived on the hill in a big house at one time, on the same street with Kobe Bryant before he was married. The first basketball game me and my sons went to was with the tickets that Kobe Bryant gave us—they were very good seats at the Forum Center. His mother and sister were friends that also utilized our services. When my mother died, this was a loss for me and my sibling, but it was a bigger loss for Jacques. His only uncle, Chris, who died prior to my mother, was now gone. His wife was lost to divorce and his kids were not there. His mother had gone abroad, and he was trying to cope and survive the attacks.

My son came for my mother's burial. As a matter of fact, I came to understand that my son was there at my mother's passing and that was very comforting for me to know he was one of the last people to see her alive at her bedside. He was around when they took her body to Africa. He went with me to do the native burial of my mother to be laid to rest next to her husband. Then we returned back to Los Angeles. He would blame himself and be incredibly sad when sober. His behavior around his ailing grandmother was traumatic for her.

Back in Los Angeles after the burial, there was a big void and he did not know how to feel. He would go out and again use methamphetamine. I plunged into work. I had not seen my two grandchildren since I returned to Los Angeles. His ex-wife made the choice to not reach back out to me despite how much she knew I loved the children, and how much she knew those children looked forward to seeing me. Her older brother had died suddenly, and he had been a rock and stood in for her, essentially with the children when my son hadn't been there. I did not want to add to her stress, especially with the ups and the downs and the revolving door with my son. I didn't want anything to upend whatever peace she had.

I knew and believed that my prayer would do more for her and the children than any physical presence at that time. I cried for them daily. I'd always loved her. I decided to try to support my son to heal and battle this brain disease that was trying to destroy our lives. I was confident that she had strong family support and friends. I knew all the grandparents were also loving and always willing to help her out. I knew that all I needed to do was trust in the Lord. The Lord would help me. The Lord has been a mighty warrior, and has kept my son alive, and the Lord has kept my life to carry the gospel and to help other people survive this illness.

Daily I humbly asked the Lord to direct me and help me hold no grudges or animosity against family or anyone. The greatest gift the Lord gave me, I believe, is the revelation of the holy spirit, to understand that he is a mighty warrior, and he is able to help me overcome both the physical attack and the oppression to keep me down. The Lord placed some strategic people in my life who will not be bought and who knew me for decades and understood the scheme of the enemy against me and my kids to rob them of their future. I was already well-rounded in Santa Monica and the West Side, even before a lot of the people moved into Santa Monica in West Side. So there was a good track record of who I was, and the attempt to throw dirt at me did not stick. The power of the Lord was at work. God, the Lord, who sees the heart of all man and understood the intent. He's the one that gets his last word.

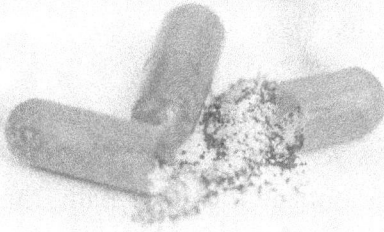

# Chapter 8

A s I learned more about substance use disorder, it became very obvious to me that drug use is very entrenched in the American culture. I never knew anyone who ever used any form of substance. My dad, after the military, started to smoke cigarettes. This was a habit that affected him, and my mother eventually died from end-stage lung disease from secondary smoke from my father's smoking even though she never smoked a cigarette in her life. She still died at the age of eighty-four, but I believe she could have lived into her nineties, just like my older sister who is still alive at the age of ninety-four.

Substance use is a brain disorder in most cases. However, there are some drug use which is just kids experimenting. This, we need to stop. Hence, the genetic predisposition that causes the brain to malfunction is triggered by environmental factors and enforced by social cultures and economic factors that allow the substance to be within easy reach of people whose ability to abstain is greatly impaired. A person who is experiencing a lot of deep pain with no outlet or other way to heal will look for ways to self-medicate. The medication from the street or pre-scription provides very quick relief and even a few good euphoria that camouflage this deep pain, then the brain triggers this cycle of wanting more and more relief.

My son would say to me, "I liked the way I felt on meth. It made me feel good. It made me feel strong. I felt like I could jump over a building many times." He has tried to jump over a building or jump heights, but for the grace of God, people came to his rescue. There was this constant need to self-destroy. Then when he's using, he will hear voices telling him to jump or hurt himself. Thank God for the police who would pick him up and transport him to a hospital where he would get treatment and hydration. Then he would experience another trigger that reminded him of his family and the loss of people he loved deeply and feeling that deep void would push him on the street again.

We know now that the quantity of meth use and frequency of use determines the symptoms and the behavioral prob-lem, as well as the physiologic problems associated with the disease. Acute psychosis, the result in multiple emer-gency room visits from use. Methamphetamine results in total body inflammation affecting primary organs. But most importantly, it affects the brain and the heart.

Many times, they will show up in the emergency depart-ment with heart attacks, brain bleeds, and many are dead on arrival. In the last two years in America, the death rate has greatly increased from methamphetamine use espe-cially when it's mixed with opioid. When I would observe my son struggle, his heart rate was faster than normal. He would occasionally complain of chest pain and physical pain in his abdomen and his bones. He had pain in his teeth due to poor dental care with tooth breakage because of extremely poor self-care and total abandonment of himself to the disease. At worst, he would refuse to listen to cooperate with any logical counseling. On methamphetamine, he saw the world backwards and even hated to be around people.

My son is a gentle giant normally and has real compassion and caring for people. He would go anywhere and give away the last shirt on his body to help someone who needed it. He is highly responsible, and if you want anything done, you can put my son to it and he will get it done correctly. When he didn't know something, he would go to Google. He would become so good at using Google to self-educate. He has a huge heart and a great presence. And as his mother, I think I know him and his brother very well. I live my life around family, helping them to be the best, the men that I believe they could be, encouraging them to learn the ways of Jesus Christ.

In fact, before we moved to Palisade High, me and my sons read the Bible daily. I believed that while I was still able to influence their lives, that the great gift I could give them, or anyone else for that matter, was a proper foundation in the word of God. They were growing up to be decent men who knew Jesus Christ and respected the law of the land. Then suddenly, this evil called methamphetamine came into our lives, and I found myself chasing the understanding of this surreal danger and harm to my boys. I did not know what it was or how to help them.

By nature, I'm a very shy person who says very little and believes in leading by example. Also, I wanted to remain their mother and that bed of comfort for them, not their disciplinarian. I was grounded in the church, and, in the church, there were leaders who were great examples of how they needed to grow into strong men and to build their own families. As time went along, I realized that my first son had leadership quality, but he wanted to play football. Mainly, he was not following the business suit or the pastoral route. The pastors at that time were former football professional players, so I was happy that he would be able to get the right counseling and excel in this area as well.

When people are dealing with deep emotional pain and rejection, it affects every area of their lives. I was deeply immersed in the program of the church. We were involved in the global church planting, and I supported the pastoral vision and went to all the places I could while also practicing medicine. I did not want my boys to be mama's boys. I felt they needed to be stand up men for their community and family.

By the time I was fifteen years old, I was already helping my parents take care of my siblings—making their food, sewing their clothes, and doing all errands for the family. When I came to America at a young age, I came alone with one suitcase. I found my college by myself, all the way from West Africa, and soon I realized that I wanted an American education. And then, as an undergraduate, I went to work in a commercial laundromat and was getting paid $2.75 folding large hospital sheets through a hard roller press. Because I learned to fear God early in my life, from my parents' teaching and watching their lives, I was confident and never fearful in a new country. For my first son, I expected no less. I was not willing to mother him to stupidity and most of the correction, as they became teenagers, I left to the pastors in the church.

When my son got kicked out of the church, he no longer had the pastoral covering. But at the time he was in a big university program at UCLA and he was by himself and had no guidance.

The substance use made him feel invincible, except he was still not getting playing time on the field. No one would help him except God. He did not understand any of these issues he was around. A lot of people are very lonely. The pastor who would have taught him to do whatever position they gave him was no longer in his life. The coach who could have directed him to this ability at the university, through his academics, did not see him regularly enough. And I essentially had lost him to the struggle to play football the only way he knew.

The life that he was brought up in was one of community with the church. Once you were of age, you would meet your wife or husband, or the pastors would help you meet someone. All of that had gone out of the window for Jacques. His first girl and puppy love in the church was now snatched away with no way to restore it. His former friends in the church were given specific instructions never to talk to him or deal with him. This was personally really difficult for Jacques to cope with. So the love and emotional support that he had was gone from the church of Jesus Christ. The counseling of God that he would normally get was gone. He was pushed away. Only love heals, and only love and the truth heals people when they have medical problems and brain disease, isolation, tough love, or ostracization does not help this problem. If anything, it compounds it and it brings despair, and this is why some of these people tend to not survive.

It was clear the young Black man in majority white churches was never accepted into the clique. They were sure the pastor always meant well for his flock and being a very conservative law-and-order kind of person, I always took the pastor's side. I was never raised to see anyone from the color of their skin. Hence, I encouraged my kids to trust the Lord and obey the pastor. It was never clear whether the pastor understood my suffering, even before the 9/11 targeting. And after that, he would often try to justify his treatment of me and my kids with very minor issues of me trying to help my fellow African who asked for help when we visited Sierra Leone for a medical mission trip. It was very hard for him to ever find anything he could say I ever did wrong to anyone. I accepted that, whatever he said.

Any help I needed to give the local people should have been through their pastor. But one of those innocent mistakes that was held over my head was that I was obedient to the pastor. It was not like somebody told me not to do anything or that I did it against the pastor's advice. It was just that they asked me for money, and I gave what I had on me. I was just trying to help the situations I saw.

In the church in Santa Monica there was some level of bias there. They forgot the years I stood with them and supported the church and the work of the kingdom as a Black person in a city where there was less than a handful of Black physicians, let alone a Black woman physician. I continued in prayer every morning at six and in church three times weekly for every church event, I asked the Lord to always help me to be humble and to follow the pastor's direction as I always respected him.

Anyway, when Jacques had his own kids, I knew that the Lord had given me a future and I hope that no matter the plan of the devil, that my God lives. Because of the rejection from the mother of his kids and their family, my son would say to me, "I thought that love was eternal." I would say, "Yes, love is forever. If it was true, it will not die. But the Love of Jesus Christ is the only one that never dies." Then my son would say, "Why couldn't she still love me when she understood that my brain is ill?" And I would say, "She is a young woman and could not understand. You need to pray for healing for you and them. You need to try to stop." But it wasn't something he could stop. He needed treatment and structure and help to stop the drug use.

It was, for him, like a huge iron press coming down on his head with no escape. For me, my grandchildren needed to be protected from the ravages of these changes and battle with addiction. I never pushed for any grandparent rights, as my daughter-in-law had to battle too much emotional trauma. I left it all to the Lord. I believed that the Lord saw me and he would get the glory in the end.

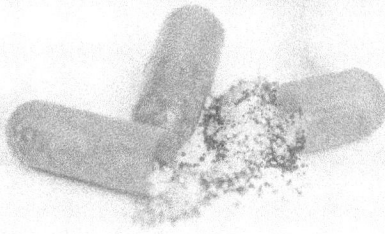

# Chapter 9

For kids who have grown up in the church, it's important to know that the church is not the protection for you if you are not obeying the commandment of the Lord. The commandment of the Lord is the only umbrella that protects you if you work under it in truth. So for children who grew up in the church, that does not mean that they will not use drugs or fall prey to the ills of the world.

Parents need to look out for any signs of depression and loss of interest in normal daily activities. Are your kids hanging out with kids you don't know or have even seen before? Are they staying away from their regular friends? Is there any big upheaval in their lives that pushes them or triggers depression and anger? Are they failing in areas where they were normally excelling? Are they hiding things from you and preferring to stay in their rooms and on computers? Are they refusing to do their homework? And is the teacher telling you they are not participating in school or not showing up to class? Have you smelled cigarette smoke or marijuana on their clothing? Do they fly off into argument and rage with you over simple issues? Do you think they are having sex or spending time with sexually explicit materials like porn?

Yes, even in church, these kids are experimenting, as teenagers, as young adults, and even the pastors' kids right under their own roof.

Are they sleeping a lot, and even the alarm clock does not wake them up? Are they lacking interest in going to school? Are they secretive about everything? A well-adjusted child or teenager should be eager to get to school at least to meet with their friends. They should be eager to tell you about school, at least if you are engaged with them and have built a level of trust and not judgment. Remember that teens are discovering their sexuality, and they see and notice and hear about everything from social media. Even if you don't allow them to use these devices, their friends will tell them. Every person, not just kids, wants to have friends and be liked by their friends. Teens and young adults do not have the level of maturity in their brain to accurately differentiate what is likely to be a danger down the line. You as their parent can see ahead to some degree and help guide them if you are engaged. *Do not allow social media to raise your kids for you.* If you are too busy or want to be your kid's friend rather than a parent, then you are likely to have a lot of regrets and painful experiences as they get more involved in worldly activities.

I need to give you one important piece of advice, especially parents of girls, though this advice is applicable to boys as well. The one area of sin that will surely destroy people's lives is sex. Even the Bible says that while most sin is outside your body, the sin of sex is deep in your body and involves your soul (1 Corinthians 8:18). If you teach your children nothing else, you must teach them how to manage their sexual behavior and new discoveries about sex with great care. If you don't have open communication with your kids about sex, a lot of pain will come home to you and them. From broken hearts to unwanted pregnancies, to sexually transmitted diseases, to HIV, to hepatitis, and drugs. Can kids enjoy life without focusing so much on sex? Yes, very much so. Help them discover the beauty of nature, from learning about birds and butterflies, to the clouds, to the weather and why things are the way they are. These are incredibly fun, beautiful things that God gave man. If you allow them to watch TV, let it be about nature and discoveries of different cultures. Teach them service to other people. Even getting out two hours every weekend on a family walk to pick up garbage in your neighborhood will allow you to meet your neighbors and discover something about them. Your very life might depend on these discoveries. You might even discover there is a kid looking for friends who do not hang with bad crowds.

There are always early signs of trouble for young kids and young adults. For the teens who have already tried drugs or have been pressured by their peers, you'll notice some of the signs that they are up to no good. For instance, they come home later than the time you give them. Take notice of their grades and how they're doing in school. Are their grades slipping? Listen to the stories they tell you. Did they share a story about how their boss at work was complaining that they did something wrong? They were very reliable kids when they were hired, but now something has changed. Are your kids wanting to spend times at friends' houses that have lesser supervision because the parents are at work or are absent for another reason?

Does the kid start losing interest in going to church? And you can tell they're having sex and using harsh language inappropriately. They want to go to parties, not in a home backyard, but in underground clubs. The underground clubs are a death trap full of drugs and sex. Your children may have never seen these behaviors before. They are now teenagers seeing everyone of various sexes having sex in the open underground clubs. The young adults will approach your teens in clubs knowing they are green and probably don't really know anything. They are virgins. Most of the times they are adults in their twenties now approaching your teenage kids of same sex to solicit sex under the influence of drugs. Maybe they just tried one type of drug and are now initiated. While my son was not going to these underground clubs in his twenties, I can't say he hasn't been to one. He was mostly just looking for acceptance. He wanted family more than anything, and he understood that as his mother, my total pursuit is the way of Jesus Christ. Would I say I did everything right? No, but I know my sons always saw this unflinching ability to stand up for the truth even if it meant denying myself of people's love. I can look in the mirror and say that since I left my husband, I have never allowed any weird person to touch my body, which is the temple of the holy spirit. I wish I knew these things in my early college days in America. My boys understood that even when they don't see me, I'm pursuing the ways of truth.

What should you do when you are convinced that your kids are engaging in activities unbecoming of your core values and beliefs? Our children and teenagers are so influenced by outside sources. People can force a lifestyle on your kids and turn them against their core values and beliefs, which are positive, healthy, and based in faith. But know this: parents, you are not helpless. Bring in help from wherever you can. Ask God on your knees what to do. He is always there to help all of us. Find out what the word of God says about children and sexuality. The Bible is a complete manual for life, so let no one fool you. Did it ever cross your mind that people outside will force a different lifestyle on your children from the way that they were raised. Did it ever occur to you that everything is by design the way things are in America and that the dollar is behind every action and every law?

Love your children enough to correct them with love. Let your children know that relationships need to be taken very seriously. You cannot allow anyone to touch your body anywhere, not in clubs and not in the home. The old adage that nothing good happens after midnight is even more true now more than ever. For your girls, nothing good happens after 10:00 p.m. You assure yourself that you will not be that parent who gets the call to come identify your kids in the morgue. Why do so many girls fall victim in America to crimes and homicide? It's not brain science. The young girls begin using alcohol because they don't think it's drugs and they want to fit in. But please remind your girls that everyone metabolizes alcohol differently. For some people, all it takes is one glass of wine and their judgment of reality is impaired enough where you are following someone away from safety without really knowing it. Alcohol is the socially accepted source of most dangers for kids and young adults, especially girls. It is also associated with several diseases, but that is a whole different book.

Intervene and get in your kid's face. I wish I knew then what I know today. Parents, you don't have to make any of these stupid mistakes for your children—that is why I'm writing this book. Thank God for His word otherwise I would have fared worse. The pursuit of the American dollar and giving away my energy and money to people who do not care about anyone it would have been better to scale down my lifestyle and give my family more than that world out there. It cost $1,000 for cocktail parties for political people who get to Washington and see that the system is so hard to change and even their best intentions can do little. They are better off praying for God to change them, as only He can do so. Maybe it would be better for private foundations to take on these difficult problems for the families and the communities.

Intervene for your children with everything you have when you can. Do not allow them to brow beat you, especially if you're a single mom. This is why the older Black women in America have great kids because they would not stand for nonsense, and neither will the Jewish families. They will learn the word of God whether they like it or not. The book of Deuteronomy tells the parent to teach His word to their children and for that they will receive generational blessings. How about you and your kids read Deuteronomy 28 as well as Exodus 20. It's not only about having the word of worldly knowledge, but you can get that in all kinds of books. It's about following the Word of God that is associated with promise and covenant for generations to come.

You cannot tie up your children in the house, but you must first educate yourself. You must know that when the kids first use drugs, they are most likely using alcohol, marijuana and/or smoking cigarettes. That would usually stick with them for a few months, even years. Their grades will slip, and they usually just get tardy and sloppy in everything. They might even go off to college. In college, they drink more and have weekend parties in the dorms.

Sometimes the colleges look the other way. The kids in sports have to meet the code of conduct. Hence their coach quickly will see these changes and try to help them. For kids not in sports, they are usually wanting to excel in academics. They will transition to "good grade" pills, like Adderall, which is approved by the FDA to treat ADHD. For the kids, these stimulant drugs have become a greatly abused drug on college and university campuses. The drug will help them be hyper-focused to study so they can pass their exams. Once the student passes the exam, they'll want to do it again. You are the parent, don't keep giving them cash and credit cards to use for whatever they want. From there they advance into harder stimulants like methamphetamines that help them to perform sexually better on college campuses and in society at large.

Please know that any time when you are not in your children's face, the dealers are in their faces with drugs like candy. They give young kids and young adults these feel-good euphoria and great sex. It does not take a brain surgeon to see that these evils naturally draw the children like magnets. A lot of the kids want to live in college dorms or homes around colleges to stay far away from the eyes of their parents and families. I was clueless and would have remained so if my grandchildren didn't come along and God allowed me the opportunity to spend time helping to raise them. The good thing about babies and young kids is that they are levelers. They brought me down to earth. Also, I did not want anything to cause them pain. And then there was my daughter-in-law whom I did not want anything to cause her pain or unhappiness especially coming from my son.

You as a parent need to know that Adderall is a stimulant like amphetamine. Even though most Adderall can be obtained by prescription, people who want to abuse it have been filling their Adderall prescriptions over the internet. But what we know now is that everything has been compromised with other drugs like fentanyl. So amphetamine combined with alcohol or heroin or OxyContin is very lethal. These drugs bind to the same receptor in the brain and displaces the natural body dopamine and floods the brain with dopamine. This is the feel-good euphoria the kids crave and go back for more. The kids who have found methamphetamines are now able to combine the feel-good euphoria with hypersexuality and they seek to sleep and have sex with anyone who even smiles at them. These drugs have increased HIV and sexually transmitted diseases and hepatitis in the cities and in the United States and world at large. The FDA has not approved any medicine to treat methamphetamine use disorder. Stimulant overdose or overuse is everywhere. It used to be that people who lived in the West were very into methamphetamine use while those in the East were big on heroin and opioid use. But now opioids and stimulants are all over the US.

In America and in society, we have a massive proliferation of these drugs in the street. You need to look for sores or needle tracks on your kid's body. They might have started with smoking and snuffing. But the quicker, feel-good euphoria is with the injectables. When they put those drugs with a needle into their bloodstream, the rush is immediate, and death is also immediate within minutes if they are alone when doing these drugs. Sometimes the needles have been used and reused, and they are very dirty and unsanitary.

You can fool yourself and think they know better than to use needles other people have used. That would be like using condoms other people have used. I can tell you that methamphetamine knows no morals, and all the user wants is to be high right there and then.

When you start missing money in your purses and your kids were by the house, it's not the Black neighborhood kid who stole your money; it's your kids who stole your money. They probably stole the money to feed their drug habit that you know nothing about. Yes, your "good" kids are drug thieves. There is absolutely nothing good that comes from the drug culture. The kid you thought you knew is no longer that person because these drugs change the brain structure and their behavior is totally different. It's only a matter of time before the police come knocking at your door.

Some of these drug dealers who do not even use drugs are becoming multimillionaires at your children's expense and on your pocketbook. The kids don't have much money. So your money is feeding the drug habits. Please do not fool yourself into thinking this is a problem "over there" or only problems for university and college kids. No, the problem is in all walks of life now in America. Drug use has greatly affected productivity and caused economic decline in America. From Wall Street to Main Street to all boardrooms to political rooms and all manners of organization, it's now clear why lots of jobs are shipped out to cultures where you can still get workers who are not under the influence of substances, be it alcohol or otherwise.

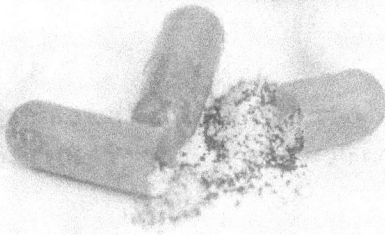

# Chapter 10

I will define for you what freedom is in a few sentences, but first I want to tell you what freedom is not. Freedom is not the ability to be able to tell yourself STOP even when your behavior affects the life of other people adversely. What would your parents and family members have given to not have your kids, brothers, and sisters come back in body bags? Would you not have denied yourself everything so they could have healing? So this is not freedom; this is a death trap camouflaged to the kids as freedom.

How will you feel when you get that dreadful call about your child's death or open the door to let the police officer in? I bet you a million dollars that you would rather to have been the bad parent protecting your kids from a life of evil and darkness than being the "everything is okay" parent. We must all take some responsibility, whether it's the kids and young adults making bad decisions, or the parents who allowed them the environment of too much freedom to adopting a selfish focus and feel-good mentality, even when there was no clear reason other than just foolish indulgence. For kids with brain disease, the street is not who should be treating them. There are enough well-trained professionals who can intervene for us and help us.

I ask myself daily what I should have done different to help my son that would have helped him enjoy his beautiful family and not have to battle these brain diseases. But I was doing everything to make everyone else better but my own kids. The responsibility squarely rests with me.

My son was living with perpetual pain. The Lord had mercy, and my son is alive. But let's be clear, it's not because I did anything right. It was by the total grace of God that my son is alive today. Even given the clear proof that my son has suffered this brain disease for many years, I should have intervened sooner. Obviously, I cannot tell you today that if I did not travel outside of the country and instead was babysitting my adult son if that would have made any difference, but I would at this point have felt that I was always there.

I blame myself, asking why he had to suffer so long. And if getting him help earlier would have helped him and his family and saved my daughter-in-law the headache. Losing my home was so traumatic for me, and the only way I knew to survive was to trust God and pivot into something else to regain control of my life.

What is freedom? Freedom is "you shall know the truth, and the truth shall make you free." The words of Jesus Christ. Freedom is knowing the truth of who Jesus Christ is and living that life in your everyday being and teaching it to your children and family. "You shall love the Lord your God with all your heart and all your mind and all your soul and with all your strength. And you shall love your neighbor as yourself." (Mark 12:30–31, NKJV) On these two commands the law rests.

Think about it. The truth is that the word of the Lord has not changed in generations. The more we live, the more we see that the flesh has not offered us much life but death. There are only temporary highs and mostly lows unless you hide yourself in His commands.

Outside of the COVID deaths, drug and alcohol contributes to 200,000 deaths of mostly men in America. This is the family destruction that no one is wanting to talk about. When I returned to Los Angeles after serving the people of California in the COVID frontline in Porterville as the Chief Medical Officer for my deployment period in the alternative care service, I learned that one of the church elder's precious son had died suddenly of drug overdose in the bathroom of their home. I was so sad and heartbroken for the family because I know them well. I watched his children grow up. Not only did we go to church together, but they lived two streets over from when I first lived in the Mar Vista area.

I had been gone from the church long, but I had recently seen his mother when I stopped at the church to say hello and see a visiting pastor. What did the parents miss? It is always easier for the church people to point out the kids who were seen as the "bad kid." Most of the time, those kids look the part with tattoos and the like. They were usually minority kids; they were kids who were in the world. They were kids who did not know God. They were kids from broken families. These were all lies and myths that people believe by and live in this bubble of deception and bias.

One of the many truths the pastor once told me and my son was, "The devil is not just trying to hurt you, he is trying to kill you." How true that is. People think they are fighting flesh and blood. People are running to the bank and taking advantage of the ignorance of the American parents about the agenda to rob them. No, it's not people who look different, that is your problem. First look in the mirror and see these spirits that we have no control over that overtake our lives.

We know for sure that many of these children have two parents in the home, parents with good education and good jobs, who have money, and who live in good neighborhoods. But these children are still involved in illegal activities that have taken their lives. Why? They are not happy. The lies they see, even from their own parents, is tormenting.

People of faith should try to live the commands of Jesus Christ. Nobody liked Zacchaeus in the Bible because he stole money from moms-and-pops in tax collection, but the Lord went to dine with him. Most "nice" people in that era never associated with the Samaritan people—the woman at the well was one such person. She was a sinner by all self-righteous standards. She was married many times, but the Lord chose her to reveal some eternal truths. "God is a Spirit and those who worship Him must worship Him in Spirit and in truth." (Joshua 4:24, ESV) Now we know the Lord is everywhere at every time, and the Lord can use anyone to accomplish His eternal objectives. We need to wake up and stop the hate. We need to stop the drugs. Maybe the lifestyle of the gay man or woman is not your way, but at no point in the Bible does it say you need to attack them physically or with your words or deny them anything or discriminate against them. The disciple of Jesus Christ is called to teach all that Christ taught them. The knowledge of God is by revelation after hearing the word delivered in love.

The Lord did not send anyone to attack people because they did not believe what you believe or live your lifestyle. Only love changes people. We need to change the way we think. People are sitting in the pews of churches for years full of hate, pride, and demons. Which God are they serving?

The myth of skin color and the economic disaster it has yielded in America is no longer acceptable. The fact is that we all have to come together to help our young people survive. When kids are properly supported by older adults in their community, they do much better. When families are properly educated about this society's evils and don't assume that evil has a color code or zip code, people can better cope with life's problems. I frequently see church people who want to go to Africa and teach people how to live, and they will not lift a finger to help the poor people in their community or in their backyard. Instead, they prefer to warehouse them and incarcerate them in private prisons. They are feeding the merchants of private prisons with your children's lives while you as a taxpayer make them very wealthy. My friends, this ought not to be so.

The decline in America will continue unless we all wake up. The world belongs to God, and this world is a journey in preparation for eternity. If we collect all the accolades and money this world has and lose our soul or our children, what benefit do we have?

Christianity is not politics and not blue and red. No political party can save us or our families. Let us have compassion for the children and young adults who have never been taught the truth or learned that the fear of the Lord is the beginning of wisdom. Kids buy into this concept: "If it feels so good, how can it be bad?" But this is wrong. This thinking that the young people have bought into is a death trap. It is nothing but a temporary high with a lifetime of misery, and worst of all, a death to hell, which is a real place.

The prostitute Rahab, who lived in the wall of Jericho, was not a believer, and neither was she a Jew. But she had one piece of critical knowledge: that the Lord of the Spies Joshua and Caleb and the men who went with them was a really powerful God and had delivered His people from great waters and carved a path where there was no path in the bottom of the sea. With this knowledge she went about orchestrating a plan to protect the spies from certain death if they were discovered. So Rahab cleared the path for God's plan and participated in the plan of God for the Messiah to come to redeem man from eternal damnation. She was not schooled in anything, but she was paying attention and told herself that the God who can do such amazing things could help her too. So she negotiated the deal of eternity. "Swear to me by The Lord that since I have shown you kindness that you also will show kindness to my father's house and give me a true token, and spare my father, my mother, brothers and my sisters and all that they have, and deliver our lives from death." (Joshua 2:12-13, NKJV) It was an eternal deal that not only saved her and her house but all who shared her blood forever.

This one critical understanding saved not just Rahab's life, but all the people who were related to her, such that almost three thousand years after that event, you are still reading about her courage. Yet many great people in the eye of men have come and gone and are forgotten by history. Rahab, a prostitute, whom no one thought much of, had cleared a path for the purpose of the Lord to be realized because God uses people. She became the great-great-great-grandmother in the human lineage of our Savior Jesus Christ, the Messiah.

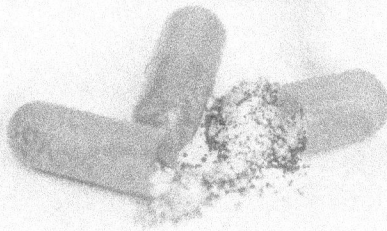

# Chapter 11

The Lord uses anyone who will humble themselves and allow the Holy Spirit to work through them for God's name to be lifted up. When the Lord called Cyrus, the King of Persia, to build the temple in Jerusalem, he was not even born for another five hundred years. He was not even a Jew. He was called by name. Maybe the proponents of abortion need to think again. The truth is that we are God's creation. Science does not contradict the Bible. In fact, the Bible told us in the Book of Daniel that we will be living the technologically enhanced life we currently live in. Daniel told us that knowledge will increase and people will go to and fro. Recent archeological discoveries in Israel unearthed the seal of the reign of King Hezekiah, as well as the prophet seal of Prophet Isaiah, who accurately predicted and described the Messiah. They amazingly lived in the same period. Even Google can tell you that.

If you ever read the Bible (and if you don't, maybe this is a good time to start) find yourself one of the greatest Bible teachers in the world, like Dr. Baruch Korman, or a great communicator and teacher like Bishop T. D. Jakes. There are many more great Bible teachers out there. These men are great communicators of the Word. So the real truth is that science eventually catches up with the Bible. For centuries, science told us that the world was flat, but the Bible already told us about the circle of the Earth in the Book of Isaiah. Over 2,500 years ago. People should not miss the opportunity to teach their children about the Bible and the full Word of God. At the very least, allow them to have this critical knowledge that could save their lives. Nowadays, people read any other junk that is out there. What do you have to lose by allowing them to read the Word of God? Let them grow up having the knowledge that there's something bigger than themselves and everyone and everything.

So now, slowly, we are seeing the world turn in our very face, in our generation and bringing the words of the Lord in the Bible more and more to the forefront. My son said to me, "When I'm walking with the Lord, I feel much better and much more at peace." Many kids find themselves lost in the world. They are looking for authenticity and grounding and adults who really care. All they hear and see are horror stories in the media. No wonder they are filled with fear, anxiety, and depression. Oh, before we forget, let's give them more drugs and the big pharmaceutical companies can run all the way to the bank. How much is enough of what you cannot even take with you? You will take not a single penny. We were told by the Egyptians that their important people needed to be buried with all kinds of treasure so that when they come back to life, they will continue to live in the manner they were accustomed to living. But we now know that this is not so. But we also see countless lives transformed by the knowledge of Jesus Christ. We also know in other religions where there is a since of focus and community there is not a lot of drug problems. Family and education are encouraged and thus allows the children to survive difficult periods in life.

The Lord is able to use what the devil meant for bad for His greater purpose. This might be an opportunity for America to clean up and rise up. A chance for the merchants of death to go into educational businesses to teach kids that drugs are wrong for their body and their brain. And even get contracts to do so. Maybe they can partner with the industry to build better transportation systems, better smart homes, and better agricultural systems so that people are not just eating unhealthy processed foods.

The Lord can use anyone, and the Lord can frustrate the agenda of evil for His greater plan of the Kingdom.

Daily I tell the Lord, "The more I know you, the more I fear you." The devil designed for me to be a bag lady, walking the streets in their wicked human experimentation, but the Lord is a great God and had another purpose for allowing this great trial in my life. Yes, the brain disease my son is recovering from will now allow your sons and your daughters to survive these wicked, evil drugs.

So how are we treating substance use disorder for kids and adults battling opioid disorder. We have had great success with methadone due to its daily dosing oral pills. The DEA has added treatment for opioid use disorder with

Suboxone, mostly sublingual, which is a film that dissolves under the tongue quickly. We also have success with naltrexone and Vivitrol, an oral pill or monthly injection. To start some of these medications, you need to be opioid use-free for a few days. You need to be off any street drug for about seven days before you can start. There has been the myth that if you allow drug treatment in your nice neighborhood, you will lower property values and attract drug use. What we see is the exact opposite. The drug treatment cut down HIV, hepatitis, and other sexually transmitted diseases in the communities.

We see that the overuse of the emergency resources is reduced, especially hospitals beds. We see reduction of crime in neighborhoods. It does not matter your zip code; untreated and unchecked proliferation of drug use will come to your zip code. It's only a matter of time. Maybe you have not read Isaiah 26:5-6, KJV, it says, "He brings down those who dwell on high, the lofty city, he layeth it low, he layeth it low to the ground and brings it down to the dust. The foot shall tread it down, the feet of the poor, and the steps of the needy."

So for right now, we see people with housing needs on the street. Unless we change how we see these deep social problems from both sides of the aisle, the day will come when they will not just come by your street but will come into your house, sleep on your bed, and where you chase the dollar, which is never enough. When you walk down the street in your Armani suits and walk over human beings sleeping in ungodly conditions on the street of your cities and consider them trash. Our problem is that God does not see them as trash, and He gets the last word. If we all give a little bit, the drug problem in our communities and in our country greatly becomes manageable and will eventually just become like another form of the diabetes management problem. There will be better control of crime in our society and police and law enforcement is not dumped on and criticized for the evil of a few. Whatever the problem is, the future for our grandchildren will be better managed. Families should not have to sell or mortgage their home to get mental care for their children or families. This is not a political issue. This is a human issue.

The high level of anxiety and fear associated with substance use needs to be properly managed. Again, I believe the church and nonprofit organizations would provide better stable management for substance use disorder. Religious and faith-based organizations should be able to help us better manage this drug and displacement of people proliferating problem. For-profit rehabilitation and incarceration in private jail is not a solution. There is no real incentive for these profit institutions to provide durable care.

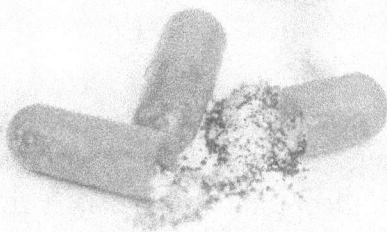

# Chapter 12

It is important to note that methamphetamine, opioid, opiates, Adderall, marijuana, heroin, OxyContin, Oxycodone, cocaine, and fentanyl are not the only drugs on the street. While these are the most common drugs, there are others that parents need to know about, such as ecstasy, bath salts, the oxymorphone a.k.a. Opana, and Molly. There are a few other concoctions that drug dealers mix in their homes and then sell to people on the street who have no money and are desperate for their next high.

It is always best for families to be involved in finding out what is causing their kid's pain. Even if your child is an adult, you as their parent still have their best interest in mind, especially when their cognition is impaired. Do not leave your child to random people because they have degrees on the wall. Help them navigate this extremely hard time until they stabilize.

One of the best indicators that something is wrong can be shown in someone's eyes. Even if you have no medical training, focus on your kid's eyes. You can tell a lot about a person by their eyes. What is the size of pupils? Are the pupils dilated? Depending on what your kid is taking, their eyes can give a quick clue that you may need to get professional help to get them through the danger zone. It is my belief that it is by the grace of God and through the commitment to the truth and commitment of money and denying myself of so much, that is the only reason I am alive today.

We all have to commit to eradicating this problem of drug abuse. The Lord has allowed my son to be alive. I will speak the Word of the Lord into his heart every day and remind him of his kids and their mother who do not deserve this to be their legacy. I will encourage him, I will build him up, and I will tell him who he is in Christ Jesus.

I tried my best to overcome whatever obstacles were placed in front of me to help my son focus on prayer and to trust in God. Through his fears and anxiety, his life has been taken over by evil things and demonic schemes that he cannot control. It has been a money pit, but what amount of money can a person place on a life redeemed by the grace of God? I know my son has skills he can use to serve God and to help other people get better from this disease. No one said it would happen overnight. But the Lord who gives people purpose, the Lord who is able to soften hardened hearts toward him, and the Lord who can reveal the truth to someone who did not fully understand his years of suffering is the Lord that we trust.

America is a very hard place to raise boys, especially now. The evil clamoring for their attention and life is everywhere. How much of this can the mind take? From violent movies, pornography, a smorgasbord of drugs, alcohol, marijuana, and nicotine, how much more can someone's mind handle before it is fried? Nowadays, kids are getting into negative habits and behaviors earlier and earlier. With time they become like robots with no mind. This is the ultimate game plan. You need to be informed and make sure you are giving consent for you and your kids.

Grown men need to be educated in the skill of their choice to handle new technology and make a good living to support their families. Men cannot thrive without self-respect and respect from their partners and family.

The only key to unlocking the door of healing is Jesus Christ. We don't give up. We don't tire. We don't accept giving our children to the devil. We stand on the solid ground of the finish work of the cross. You must allow the Lord to lead you and your family to where you can begin this journey. Even when all doors close in your face, the Lord himself can open doors that you did not see coming. He can use anyone to accomplish His greater objective. Even the hard-driving district attorneys, the Lord can touch their hearts and allow them to see His greater purpose in people who are deemed "throwaways." You cannot paint with a broad brush all the time. We humble ourselves so that the Holy Spirit can work with us.

It was clear to me that even the judge and the attorneys in our case came together, and in the end, they agreed on a good outcome. The Lord brought in an amazing young man named Shawn to become the brother that my son needed.

He needed to be accepted where he was. And even against all attacks from my ex-husband and my other son, I knew I would do the same for my son and his kids and stand for them. No amount of money will stop me from helping my son, as I know how he has suffered from this disease where everyone failed to intervene on a timely basis.

I cannot roll over and watch my son die from rejection after the Lord saved his life. The drug institutions are so large in this country and so full of failure, even the most hardened person is open to a miracle. This is how we got where we are today, by the grace of God.

As mentioned, there is no FDA-approved drug for treatment of methamphetamine and other stimulants use disorder, but there are people working on it. There are doctors who will not quit, and I will not quit making sure that you, as parents, get the truth. We can only now treat with what we call Contingencies Management (CM) with reward programs and education. When people fully understand the danger to themselves, they are more likely to work harder and more over, when they know the harm they can unknowingly do to others for lack of knowledge they are more eager to cooperate with getting care.

Methamphetamine and opioid use affect just about every organ system, but more importantly the brain and heart. This also affects anywhere there are opioid receptors, the liver, the kidneys, the gut, and even the sexual organs. The opioid suppresses the central nervous system. When someone overdoses, the respiratory centers of the brain and the lungs are mostly affected. And people die even when you think they are just sleeping. Sometimes people without knowledge are mixing drugs because they can't keep their eyes open when they're high on opioids. And with methamphetamine and stimulates they can't go to sleep. Either way, it's a death trap. They fail to understand that fentanyl is ten times more powerful and has the ability to quickly displace the methamphetamine on the receptors and suppresses their ability to breathe on their own and they die, not knowing what hit them. Families are left shattered all around the nation in the United States.

In 2021 with COVID, fentanyl, and people cooped up the in house, many deaths happened in the home and in small private parties. To be clear, methamphetamine by itself is an extremely dangerous drug. The drug itself is known to cause strokes, heart attacks, and death. The euphoria became so secondary to the lethal level of drug causing acute myocardial infarction (heart attacks), as the blood vessel or the myocardium muscles also tear. It is also not difficult to see how much methamphetamine in large doses hits multiple organ systems. Usually, users are using over years, and the damages are progressive and accumulating without knowing their lives are dangling by the thread. Then add cocaine and fentanyl into the mix and one fatal day there is nothing even Narcan can do to get them to the hospital. Similarly, people using Adderall for ADHD treatment and mixing it with alcohol have health concerns they need to know about. These people can also have very sudden myocardial events. Over time, they usually develop high blood pressure, and taking with alcohol will develop and further compromise their myocardial function. They are predisposed to sudden catastrophic myocardial event.

People who use heroin and OxyContin and adding fentanyl to it for stronger euphoria are also on very thin ice. They might see this surge of euphoria a few times while mixing, but it usually lapses into very deep central nervous system depression where they can no longer breathe for themselves. Narcan could help them if someone can get there in time. But what we see is people are going into the bathrooms by themselves or with friends who are equally stoned and ine-briated. Hence multiple deaths are happening, some at the same time, in homes and in some private parties. Another horrible situation takes place at public music events where people use mostly stimulants to enjoy the event and stay awake. They fail to understand that the stimulants are contaminated with fentanyl at various quantities. So the high-class suppliers have now become the purveyor of death. What can we say to the parents, friends, and families? One evening of fun does not have to be your last. If you're not quite sure what to do with your life at a young age, sign up for the military. They will help you fix your head, and you will be happy for it at a later time. Even your family will be happy you did something great with your life.

The problem of drug use in America is such that one book cannot do its justice. But this is just the beginning. Drug use is a major problem in the United States, and we need to educate people so we can help them better understand what the impact of one day of drug use, weeks of drug use, or even years of drugs use can do to a person's productivity.

I believe we can provide treatment for people who suffer from substance abuse disorder. I believe we can come together as a nation of all different walks of life, regardless of political affiliation, and create programs, funding, and physical, emotional, and spiritual support for people with substance use disorder, and their families, and loved ones.

I end this book by reminding parents, families, churches, synagogues, mosques, clubs, and communities, that the world has changed. It's changing very rapidly and you cannot keep up unless you educate yourself with truth and are engaged regularly.

Even if you are not a Believer in Jesus Christ, you should read the Bible and encourage your kids and families and friend to do so. This is the only source of real truth.

Jesus said, "They shall know the truth and the truth shall make you free." (John 8:32, NKJV) This is talking about freedom to see right from wrong, freedom to make correct choices and freedom from subjugation of wicked ideologies

Even if you feel the Bible does not support your current choices you should still understand that Jesus Christ is for you and died for you and desires that none of us perish.

Parents, grandparents, and guardians should encourage kids not to hate or judge people base on what they look like but based on their character. The things you do daily should build your families spirit for survival.

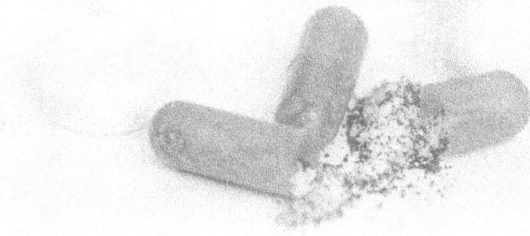

# Dedication

T he book is dedicated to my mother and father who taught me to love Jesus Christ.

To my son, Jacques, who has suffered too much from substance use disease.

To my daughter-in-law, Meghan Lazarus, an exceptional young woman whom I love dearly. To my grandchildren, Greyson and Ella Lazarus, I love you. To Gabriella Burke, Terry Burke, and all of the Burke family, thank you.

To all the pastors around the globe who have prayed for me and my family in this prolonged trial. Pastor Robert and Jennifer Scribner and Pastor Harrison and Pam Sommer.

To Dr. Baruch Korman and his wife Rifka for the amazing biblical teaching from LoveIsrael.

To my dear friends Beverly Tai, Youko Yeracaris, Jessie Sherrod, and Lillian Chew and many more who taught me what friendship meant.

To David Lazarus, my ex and forever friend and partner. I learned to forgive and obey God, and it made things better

To my sisters: Stella Nwobi, thank you. I love you. To Chioma and family, and dear Victor, I love you all. To Helen and family, I love you.

To my sister Amaka and her husband, thank you for helping me look forward.

To all the families and parents who have lost precious children to this evil, may the Lord comfort you and help you to invest your pain into saving other kids.

To my son Matthew Lazarus, keep seeking God, for he is all.

To Sarah Lazarus, Eleanor Lazarus, Isaiah Lazarus and Joshua Lazarus, I love you all. Please focus on knowing Jesus Christ as He will never leave you or forsake you.

Special thanks to Dr. Jerry Abraham who helped Jacques and I at a critical time during the COVID-19 pandemic.

Special thanks to Cynthia Ohmstead for your help with Jacques.

To Lynette Jones, thank you.

To Dionne Warwick, we will not give up.

Finally, a special thanks to Tony Robbins, Dean Graziosi, Jack Canfield, and Steve Harrison for teaching me how to turn my mess into a message to save and serve fellow human beings.

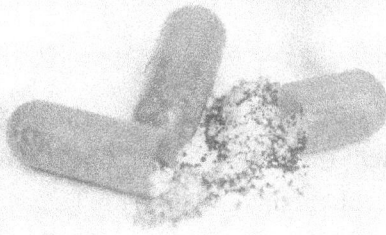

# About the Author

**D**r. Veronica A. Lazarus is a renowned health practitioner and philanthropist. She is a doctor of Internal Medicine, Emergency Medicine, Dermatology and Addiction Medicine. Early in her career doctor Lazarus was a developer of therapeutic skin care products for Dermatologist and Plastic Surgeons with her then company Galaxy Pharmaceutical. She created over three hundred different products, some for global celebrities like Dionne Warwick. Doctor Lazarus was the first to introduce Hand Sanitizer to the American Retail Market at the National Retail Show.

Dr Lazarus Practiced Medicine in Santa Monica and Beverly Hills and published research articles with Nicolas Lowe MD in prestigious journals like Journal of Investigative Dermatology, Journal of American Academy of Dermatology and Journal of Clinical Research.

In 1994 the tragedy in Rwanda was unfolding. Doctor Lazarus could not sit and just watch. She started call to the doctors in the area, including emergency room doctors, to come with her to help in Rwanda. She put together a team of thirty-seven health professionals, including pastors, to go with her to help out. After encountering many obstacles with well-established NGO, Doctor Lazarus contacted the United Nations High Commission on Refugees for assistant to get her team where help was needed.

The United Nations opened a great door that brought other help for the team. The Local hospitals like St. John's Hospital in Santa Monica, Local Doctors such as Peter Pelikan and many others came together to donate money for the team. Hence, LightHouse Doctors and Nurses International was born.

The United State Government also provided C17 Cargo Planes to get the team from the Main Air base in Germany to Goma Zaire. From there, United Nations provided two small Aircraft to take the team to Bukavu where the United Nations assigned the team. In Bukavu there were over 500,000 refugees fleeing the genocide and the journey was treacherous for the refugees, many died before getting to Zaire and safety in Bukavu. Doctor Lazarus's team quickly set up a tent hospital with the help of Canadian, British and America military men.

The Refugees poured in. One of the first refugees was a woman who had lost three children to starvation, dehydration and Kwashiorkor and marasma. She had one child hanging on her breast at the verge of death. The team was able to resuscitate the child and hand her back to her mother as her only living child. Then two weeks that turned into five months were covered by the Associated Press in September 1994. After that experience doctor Lazarus changed her whole idea about why she went into medicine. Doctors Lazarus has worked silently in the areas of medical missions and disaster for decades without accolades. At Katrina she took a team from Los Angeles to New Orleans, Barton Rouge Louisiana. The Original Non-Profit LightHouse Doctors and Nurses International was changed to Doctors and Nurses to the World Foundation in 2018.

Now this disaster was personal. Doctor Lazarus's eldest son, who has two amazing children, has substance use disorder. It is now all consuming and Doctor has once again poured in her energy to bring valuable help to parents in America to help them help their kids and families from the unspoken tragedy of Drug Addiction and Fentanyl crisis.

**She asks the question, "What will it take for America to put money into the right causes like drug addiction. How many of our kids have to die before we all respond to this crisis of our generation as a nation?"**

Doctor Lazarus earned a Master of science, Master of Art and a Doctor of Medicine degree from the State University of Buffalo School of Medical Sciences. Her MA thesis was on the Electron Microscopy of Epidermal and Dermal tissues. She completed post graduate training in Internal Medicine at The University of California Los Angeles Wadsworth VA Hospital. She also completed a two-year clinical dermatology Fellowship under Dr Nicholas Lowe at The University of California Los Angeles California. Doctor Lazarus received a scientific award for her research Work in Dermatology from The Society of Investigative Dermatology.

Doctor Lazarus built several Corporations all dedicated to raising funds for Worldwide Humanitarian Projects. Today Doctor Lazarus lives in Los Angeles and is the CEO of Doctors and Nurses to the World Foundation.

Before returning to Los Angeles she lived in China for three and half years, in Hamburg Germany, and London England for two and a half years.

Doctor Lazarus's mother passed away in 2018. It was a great loss as she had spent a lot of time trying to get Stem Cells to help her mother recover her lungs from the ravages of COPD, even though her mother never smoked a day in her life.

Doctor Lazarus's son is still battling substance use and the brain damage associated with street drugs. A huge number of prayers, resources and energy have been invested into her son's battle with substance use. The damage done to America by this demon of drugs and alcohol cannot be put into dollars and cents as it will be so huge it would blow everyone's mind. The deaths of young people in their most productive years, loss of potential and productivity goes into the Trillions. Why is this not part of our media and political dialogue? We cannot do business as usual anymore, we must respond to this evil of our time together and war against it.

Please get the book for all your friends and family. When they come back in body bags, it is too late. Your best eulogy will mean nothing. The time to Pray for America Is now.

May The Lord Get Glory in The End.

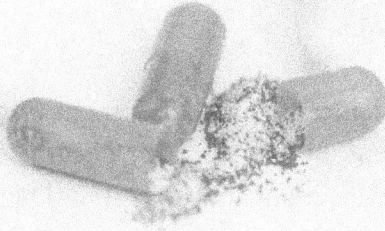

# References

Kardashian, Kim. 2019. *Prison reform and clemency advocacy.* https://en.wikipedia.org/wiki/Kim_Kardashian#Activism:

First Opioid Epidemic In America goes back to the 1620s when a physician brought the drug in his suitcase on the Mayflower (Ref National Library of Medicine. Saturday Evening Post 1885)

Ref; fending off Fentanyl and hunting down Heroin. Controlling Opioid Supply from Mexico

Opioid Crisis in America

Brooking Institute: VandaFelbab-Brown

A paper series from Foreign Policy and Global Economy and Development Program July 2020

DEA Approval of Methadone Clinic

Institute of Medicine. 1995. Development of Medications for the Treatment of Opiate and Cocaine Addictions; Issues for the Government and Cocaine Addictions; Issues for the Government and Private Sector, CE Fulco, editor; CT Liverman, editor, and LE Earley, editor., eds., National Academy Press, Washington, D.C.

SAMHSA is the lead Federal agency for public health efforts to advance behavioral health prevention, intervention, treatment, and recovery for individuals and their families.US GOV 2022

www.ingramcontent.com/pod-product-compliance
Lightning Source LLC
Chambersburg PA
CBHW072159270326
41930CB00011B/2484